Point Selection

Soothing the TROUBLED MIND

Acupuncture and Moxibustion in the
Treatment and Prevention of Schizophrenia

Translated by
Thomas Dey

Edited by
Nigel Wiseman

Foreword by
Richard Warner, PhD, DPM

PARADIGM PUBLICATIONS

BROOKLINE, MASSACHUSETTS ~ 2000

Soothing the Troubled Mind
Acupuncture and Moxibustion in the
Treatment and Prevention of Schizophrenia

Translated by Thomas Dey

Library of Congress Cataloging-in-Publication data:
Lou, Pai-ts'eng.
  [Chen chiu fang chih ching shen fen lieh cheng. English]
  Soothing the troubled mind : acupuncture and moxibustion in the
treatment of schizophrenia / translated by Thomas Dey.
      p. cm.
Includes bibliographical references and index.
  ISBN 0-912111-60-7 (pbk. : alk. paper)
  1. Schizophrenia--Alternative treatment. 2. Acupuncture. 3. Moxa.
4. Mental illness--Alternative treatment. I. Lou, Hsing-huang. II.
Dey, Thomas, 1961- III. Title.
  RC514 .L58713 1999
  616.89'8206--dc21

                              99-050641

~ Published by ~
Paradigm Publications
Brookline, MA
http://www.paradigm-pubs.com
Printed in the United States of America

ISBN # 0-912111-60-7

TABLE OF CONTENTS

ACKNOWLEDGEMENTS

P UTTING TOGETHER A BOOK is a long and involved process. If we think of the trees that are the source of paper for books, then the vast roots of a book's physical material immediately come to mind. When thinking of the origins of this book's contents, I am compelled to think of the dedicated studies, efforts, and experience of the original authors, the editor, the publishers, and many others who contributed to this publication, thereby allowing my work as a translator to reach you, the reader. There is much for me to acknowledge.

First and foremost I express my gratitude to my Buddhist Teachers. Because my Teachers are responsible for planting the seed for this work, may whatever good merit is earned hereby be dedicated to Their long lives and to the happiness of all sentient beings under the sky.

There are more reasons than I can express to thank my parents for their considerable role in this translation. They supported me while I was learning Chinese and were supportive while I was learning acupuncture (and at all times); they always encouraged me to do good things for others and always wanted me to do what I wanted to do. May they be fully pleased with this work.

In the course of going through the various drafts that culminated in this volume, there were numerous friends who helped in one way or another with various aspects of typing, word processing, computer troubleshooting, proofreading, library research, and so forth. Though I am not naming them individually here, they each have my heartfelt gratitude.

There were also many people who generously contributed their expertise to the final draft of this volume. I wish to thank Dr. Joan Cheu for her answers to questions regarding the translation of technical words in the field of psychology; her assistant, Donna Shaban, was also very helpful in reviewing the use of English psychology terminology. Dr. Chen Jian-Ping came up with clear translations of many phrases that were related to peculiar uses of psychology terminology in the PRC, many of which had left other experts simply baffled; without his contribution there could have been gaping holes in the final publication. Dr. Susan Lin, of Lin Sisters Herb Shop, also was very patient in contributing her time and understanding while explaining obscure TCM phrases. In the last stage of preparation for publication, Craig Mitchell was indispensible in clarifying how readers who are familiar with the Wiseman translation protocol (which is discussed in the Preface) would expect to see certain terms translated; he also helped with some classical Chinese phrases that I had no business trying to translate on my own. To all these people, I wish to express my gratitude three times over.

Is it possible to thank Dr. Richard Warner enough? After reading his book, *Recovery from Schizophrenia; Psychiatry and Political Economy,* it occurred to me that it would be too good to be true if he would review *Soothing the Troubled Mind* and provide some sort of an introduction to this subject. He was extremely generous in consenting to do so, and has written an introduction that gives this book, as a translation, a completeness that it would otherwise be lacking. After he worked his part of the writing into his busy schedule, there were many delays before this final publication emerged. I hope he understands how appreciative we are for what he has contributed.

From my comments in the Preface, readers can probably guess what great esteem I hold for Nigel Wiseman. One of the roots of this book is the lifetime of work that Nigel has put into developing a systematic way to translate Chinese medical literature.

Beyond that, he devoted a good deal of time and attention to reviewing, critiquing, and upgrading this volume; I frequently find myself applying some of the lessons that I learned from this great scholar even when what I am doing has nothing to do with Chinese medicine. I thank him very deeply and wish that all of his work will succeed.

Next I wish to thank Bob Felt, Martha Fielding, and everyone at Paradigm Publications who contributed their expertise and efforts to putting *Soothing the Troubled Mind* in its final form. Here again it is not just their work on this book that deserves the thanks; readers should recognize what an awesome job they have done by dedicating their lives and careers to running a publishing house that sets the standard for all other publishers of Chinese medical translations. Moreover, they have established their business in such a way that even a novice translator like myself can make a small contribution to a field where there is a vast amount of yet-to-be-done work. I look forward to working with them for many years into the future.

Finally, not wishing to obscure the forest for the trees, the last word of thanks goes to the readers. It is the readers who buy the books, read them, and apply their knowledge and experiences to understanding them. It is the readers for whom we set our standards, and who make the work of producing books worthwhile. In short, to the people who read this book and reevaluate their efforts to help soothe troubled minds: Thank you.

Thomas Dey
December, 1999

FOREWORD

THIS FASCINATING BOOK about how schizophrenia is perceived, experienced, and treated in another culture advances our understanding of one of mankind's great afflictions. As a basis of comparison, in this foreword I have set out some of what we know about schizophrenia within Western medicine.

WHAT IS SCHIZOPHRENIA?

In our own popular culture, there may be more widespread ignorance about schizophrenia than any other common illness. Ask a classroom of American college students—in engineering or English literature—what they know about AIDS or cancer and they will probably have a lot to say. But ask about schizophrenia and the silence will be embarrassing. Although schizophrenia is more common than AIDS/HIV, most people know far less about it. "Isn't it like multiple personality disorder?" people ask. "Is it caused by child abuse?" "Are they mentally retarded?" The answer to all these questions is "No."

What is it about this condition that stifles discussion and learning? AIDS, cancer, and schizophrenia are all perceived as contaminating and incurable, but somehow people with schizophrenia are seen as more mysterious, alien, and violent. Centuries of fear have promulgated many myths about schizophrenia. What are the facts?

Schizophrenia is a psychosis. That is to say, it is a severe mental disorder in which the person's emotions, thinking, judgment, and grasp of reality are so disturbed that his or her functioning is seriously impaired. The symptoms of schizophrenia are often divided into "positive" and "negative." Positive symptoms are abnormal experiences and perceptions like delusions, hallucinations, thought disorders, and disorganized behavior. Negative symptoms are the absence of normal thoughts, emotions and behavior—such as blunted emotions, loss of drive, poverty of thought, and social withdrawal.

DIAGNOSTIC DIFFICULTIES

Problems abound in defining schizophrenia. In this book, although each case illustration deals with someone who suffers from a psychosis, it is not clear that every one would be diagnosed with schizophrenia by an American psychiatrist.

The two most common functional psychoses are schizophrenia and manic-depressive illness (also known as "bipolar affective disorder"). The distinction between the two is not easy to make and psychiatrists in different parts of the world at different times have drawn the boundaries in different ways. Manic-depressive illness is an episodic disorder in which psychotic symptoms are associated with severe alterations in mood—at times elated, agitated episodes of mania, at other times depression, with physical and mental slowing, despair, guilt, and low self-esteem.

On the other hand, the course of schizophrenia, though fluctuating, tends to be more continuous, and the person's display of emotion is likely to be incongruous or lacking in spontaneity. Markedly illogical thinking is common in schizophrenia. Auditory hallucinations may occur in either manic-depressive illness or schizophrenia, but in schizophrenia they are more likely to be hallucinations commenting on the person's actions or conversing one with another. Delusions also can occur in both conditions; in schizophrenia they may give the individual the sense that he or she is being controlled by outside forces or that his or her thoughts are being broadcast or interfered with.

Despite common features, different forms of schizophrenia are quite dissimilar. One person, for example, may be paranoid but show good judgment and a high level of functionality in many areas of life. Another may be bizarre in manner and appearance, preoccupied with delusions of bodily disorder, passive and withdrawn. So marked are the differences, in fact, that many experts believe that, when the causes of schizophrenia are worked out, the illness will prove to be a set of different conditions which lead, via a final common pathway of biochemical interactions, to similar consequences.

It is not at all clear what is schizophrenia and what is not. Scandinavian psychiatrists have tended to use a narrow definition of the illness with an emphasis on poor outcome. Russian psychiatrists have adhered to a broad definition with an emphasis on social adjustment. In the United States the diagnostic approach to schizophrenia used to be very broad. With the publication in 1980 of the third edition of the *American Psychiatric Association Diagnostic and Statistical Manual,* however, American psychiatry switched from one of the broadest concepts of schizophrenia in the world to one of the narrowest.

Why is the diagnosis so susceptible to fashion? The underlying problem is that schizophrenia and manic-depressive illness share many common symptoms. During an acute episode it is often not possible to tell them apart without knowing the prior history of the illness. The records of people with manic-depressive illness should reveal prior episodes of depression and mania with interludes of normal functioning.

Schizophrenia is universal.

We should not let confusion about differentiating schizophrenia from other psychoses detract from the fact that schizophrenia is a universal condition and an ancient one. Typical cases may be distinguished in the medical writings of ancient Greece and Rome, and the condition occurs today in every human society. While the content of delusions and hallucinations varies from culture to culture, the form of the illness is similar everywhere. Two World Health Organization studies, applying a standardized diagnostic approach, have identified characteristic cases of schizophrenia in developed and developing world countries from many parts of the world.

More surprisingly, these studies have demonstrated that the rate of occurrence of new cases of the condition is similar in every country studied from India to Ireland. However, since both death and recovery rates for people with psychosis are higher in the Third World, the prevalence of schizophrenia (the number of cases to be found at any time) is lower in the Third World—around 0.3% of the population compared to about 0.6% in the developed world.

People recover from schizophrenia.

The popular and professional view that schizophrenia has a progressive, downhill course with universally poor outcome is a myth. Over the course of months or years, about 20 to 25 percent of people with schizophrenia recover completely from the illness—all their psychotic symptoms disappear and they return to their previous level of functioning. Another 20 percent continue to have some symptoms, but they are able to lead satisfying and productive lives.

In the developing countries, recovery rates are even better. The two World Health Organization studies mentioned above have shown that good outcome occurs in about twice as many patients diagnosed with schizophrenia in the developing world as in the developed world. The reason for the better outcome in the Third World is not completely understood, but it may be that many people with mental illness in developing world villages are better accepted, less stigmatized, and more likely to find work in a subsistence agricultural economy.

WHAT CAUSES SCHIZOPHRENIA?

There is no single organic defect or infectious agent which causes schizophrenia, but a variety of factors increase the risk of getting the illness—among them, genetics and obstetric complications.

GENETICS

Relatives of people with schizophrenia have a greater risk of developing the illness, the risk being progressively higher among those who are genetically more similar to the person with schizophrenia. For a nephew or aunt the lifetime risk is about two percent (twice the risk for someone in the general population); for a sibling, parent, or child the risk is about 10%, and for an identical twin (genetically identical to the person with schizophrenia), the risk is close to 50%.

Studies of people adopted in infancy reveal that the increased risk of schizophrenia among the relatives of people with the illness is due to inheritance rather than environment. The children of people with schizophrenia have the same increased prevalence of the illness whether they are raised by their biological, schizophrenic parent or by adoptive parents.

Obstetric complications

Since identical twins only have a 50% risk of developing the illness, we know that genetics alone do not explain why someone gets the illness. Other powerful factors have to play a part; one of these is problems of pregnancy and delivery. The risk for people born with obstetric complications, such as prolonged labor, is two or three times greater than for those born with none. A history of obstetric complications has been found in one third to one half of patients with schizophrenia, making it a major risk factor.

Viruses

The risk of intrauterine brain damage is increased if a pregnant woman contracts a viral illness. We know that more people with schizophrenia are born in the late winter or spring than at other times of year, and that this birth bulge increases after epidemics of viral illnesses like influenza, measles and chickenpox. Maternal viral infections, however, probably account for only a relatively small part of the increased risk for schizophrenia.

Poor parenting is not a cause of schizophrenia.

Contrary to the beliefs of professionals prior to the 1970's and to the impression still promoted by the popular media, there is no evidence, even after decades of research, that family or parenting problems cause schizophrenia.

As early as 1948, psychoanalysts proposed that mothers fostered schizophrenia in their offspring through cold and distant parenting. Others blamed parental schisms, and confusing patterns of communication within the family. The double-bind theory, put forward by anthropologist Gregory Bateson, argued that schizophrenia is promoted by contradictory parental messages from which the child is unable to escape. Although enjoying broad public recognition, such theories have seldom been adequately tested, and none of the research satisfactorily resolves the question of whether differences found in the families of people with schizophrenia are the cause or the effect of psychological abnormalities in the disturbed family member.

Millions of family members of people with schizophrenia have suffered shame, guilt, and stigma because of this widespread misconception.

Drug abuse is not a cause of schizophrenia.

Hallucinogenic drugs like LSD can induce short-lasting episodes of psychosis and the heavy use of marijuana and stimulant drugs like cocaine and amphetamines may precipitate brief, toxic psychoses with features similar to schizophrenia. It is also possible, though not certain, that while not a causative factor, drug abuse can trigger the onset of schizophrenia.

Relatives of a person with schizophrenia sometimes blame hallucinogenic drugs for causing the illness, but they are mistaken. We know this because, in the 1950's and 1960's, LSD was used as an experimental drug in psychiatry in Britain and America. The proportion of these volunteers and patients who developed a long-lasting psychosis like schizophrenia was scarcely greater than in the general population. It is true that a Swedish study found that army conscripts who used marijuana heavily were six times more likely to develop schizophrenia later in life, but this was probably because those people who were destined to develop schizophrenia were more likely to use marijuana as a way to cope with the premorbid symptoms of the illness.

WHAT WORKS?

There is more agreement now about what is important in the treatment of schizophrenia than ever before. In a recent global project designed to combat the stigma of schizophrenia, prominent psychiatrists from all around the world signed on to the following set of principles:

People with schizophrenia can be treated effectively in a variety of settings. The use of hospitals is mainly reserved for those encountering an acute relapse. Outside of the hospital, a range of alternative treatment settings have been devised which provide supervision and support and which are less alienating and coercive than the hospital.

Family involvement can improve the effectiveness of treatment. A solid body of research has demonstrated that relapse in schizophrenia is much less frequent when families are provided with support and education about schizophrenia.

Medications are an important part of treatment but they are only part of the answer. They can reduce or eliminate positive symptoms but they have a negligible effect on negative symptoms. Fortunately, modern, novel anti-psychotic medications, introduced in the past few years, can provide benefits with less severe side-effects than standard anti-psychotic drugs, which were introduced in the mid-1950's.

Treatment should include social rehabilitation. People with schizophrenia usually need help to improve their functioning in the community. This can include training in basic living skills, assistance with a host of day-to-day tasks, and job training, job placement, and work support.

Work helps people recover from schizophrenia. Productive activity is basic to a person's sense of identity and worth. The availability of work in a subsistence economy may be one of the main reasons that outcome from schizophrenia is so much better in Third World villages. Given training and support, most people with schizophrenia can work.

People with schizophrenia can get worse if treated punitively or confined unnecessarily. Extended hospital stays are rarely necessary if good community treatment is available. Jail or prison are not appropriate places of care. Yet, around the world, large numbers of people with schizophrenia are housed in prison cells, usually charged with minor crimes, largely because of the lack of adequate community treatment.

People with schizophrenia and their family members should help plan and even deliver treatment. Consumers can be successfully employed in treatment programs, and when they help train treatment staff, professional attitudes and patient outcome both improve.

People's responses towards someone with schizophrenia influence the person's course of illness and quality of life. Negative attitudes can push people with schizophrenia and their families into hiding the illness and drive them away from help. If people with schizophrenia are shunned and feared, they cannot be genuine members of their own community. They become isolated, and victims of discrimination in employment, accommodation, and education.

CAN ACUPUNCTURE AID THE PROCESS OF RECOVERY?

Within the Western medical framework outlined in this introduction, acupuncture can certainly play a role in the treatment of schizophrenia, insofar as it meets the following criteria:

~It is a less stigmatizing treatment approach than alternative forms of treatment;

~It is non-alienating, non-coercive, non-intrusive, and respects the individual and his or her personal integrity;

~It mobilizes an optimistic social consensus, is part of a vigorous effort to achieve a cure, and encourages involvement of the broader social group to aid the reintegration of the ill person. It enhances family support.

There may well be levels far beyond these in which acupuncture has a place to play in the treatment of schizophrenia.

Now read on.

Richard Warner, M.B., D.P.M.

TRANSLATOR'S PREFACE

IN INTRODUCING THIS TRANSLATION I would like to note the theme included in the authors' introduction to the original Chinese work, *Zhen Jiu Fang Zhi Jing Shen Fen Lie Zheng* (*Acupuncture and Moxibustion in the Treatment and Prevention of Schizophrenia*). The authors selected a four-character Chinese saying to describe their book that literally translates as, "Cast brick; elicit jade." When a Chinese speaker uses this saying, Chinese listeners instantly perceive the image of a crude and laborious job being done in order to ultimately develop a valuable, refined treasure. In the course of this introduction I hope to explain to Western readers why this book, which may seem hopelessly slight for the great and noble task the authors undertake, should be closely examined to find its true treasure.

During the 1980's, while living in the People's Republic of China over a period of several years, I attended a three-month session at the Nanjing College of TCM International Acupuncture Training Centre. It was an impressive experience. The main campus of the college covered a large city block. It had student dormitories, a cafeteria, an athletic field, and classroom buildings to accommodate several hundred undergraduate and graduate students, all of whom were specializing in acupuncture, herbology, therapeutic massage, and other aspects of Chinese medicine. The faculty gave students both classroom and clinical training; they conducted research, and wrote and published journals and books.

Not only was there the enormity of the surroundings, there was the enormity of the visible societal impact. Besides an entire hospital that applied primarily TCM treatments, there were also several TCM outpatient clinics, some with a daily patient load in the thousands.

Thus, while the experience of living amongst Chinese people made it clear to me that TCM is a living part of Chinese culture, studying at the Nanjing College of TCM gave me the direct and powerful experience of using Chinese medicine for treating all manner of disease. There was no question as to whether or not TCM worked. The sheer volume of patient care was enough to make it very clear that this was no experiment.

It was as a result of the considerable impression which my TCM studies had on me that I decided to undertake the translation of this specialized work. It is my strong belief that there is much suffering by people with mental diseases that could be alleviated if TCM were better understood.

Many in our post-modern Western society question whether allopathic medicine will reach the goal of curing all disease. While we respect some of the miraculous achievements of modern medicine, and rely on it in many ways, we no longer look to physicians with complete faith, and there is large-scale acceptance of various forms of alternative medicine. Within this scenario it seems obvious to me that during the 21st century a transcultural adaptation of Chinese medicine will become an influential dynamic in our native Western medical systems. It is my hope that this work will help to clear the path to such an outcome.

A NOTE REGARDING TRANSLATIONAL GOALS

My main goal in translating this book has been to provide a resource for English-speaking practitioners of Traditional Chinese Medicine (TCM), for Western-trained psychology specialists, and for individuals (and their families and friends) who suffer from mental diseases.

RESOURCES FOR ENGLISH-SPEAKING PRACTITIONERS OF TCM

For TCM specialists, this book explains a basic protocol for treating all mental diseases. It gives an historical overview of mental disease treatments, including treatments for obscure symptoms, and provides details on various ways in which the modalities of TCM have been used successfully, either uniquely or in combination with Western pharmacotherapeutic treatments.

RESOURCES FOR WESTERN-TRAINED PSYCHOLOGY SPECIALISTS

For psychology specialists, this book invites an appreciation for the complexity and usefulness of TCM. In fact, TCM has arguably its greatest utility when it is not explicated or delimited by the theories of modern allopathic disease naming and symptomatology. Thus professionals who have long worked within the confines of environmental/congenital and physical/mental debates should find it useful and renewing to have mental diseases described from a well-developed and entirely different perspective—that of yin/yang and the five phases.

Additionally, the psychology specialist can discover how TCM, or TCM in conjunction with Western medicine, is used for patients in China who have psychological disorders. For example, a full-scale Chinese treatment will be coupled with a greatly reduced dosage of an allopathic pharmaceutical drug that is either very expensive or likely to produce strong side-effects. Thus it provides a basis for psychology specialists to cooperate with TCM practitioners on the joint treatment of patients.

RESOURCES FOR THE GENERAL READER

General readers could utilize the information in this book by being aware of simple and effective treatment protocols that could be administered by their specialist or by referral. Patient involvement is a critical and acceptable tool in the quest for healing.

In aiming for this goal, the general reader will find it useful to understand the basic fourfold process of TCM. First, the practitioner collects diagnostic information by reading a patient's pulse, visually observing the patient (especially the tongue), hearing and smelling various changes in the patient, and asking a series of diagnostic questions. Based on the data observed, the practitioner subsequently selects a pattern from amongst the theories of TCM that most closely describes the underlying imbalance in the patient's health. Next, the practitioner determines the principle of treatment that should be applied to restore balance. Finally, treatment is applied to carry out the treatment principle. The treatment formulary could be the use of medicinal agents, the use of acupuncture, or the use of any ancillary TCM treatments, depending on the determination of the physician as to what treatment would most effectively carry out the treatment principle.

TCM is thus a wonderful resource. Although from one point of view mastery of TCM requires a lifetime of study and practice—an expert herbologist must learn how to combine as many as 15 or 20 ingredients from a pharmacopoeia of over 2,000 ingredients in order to be able to help patients with all manner of disease—from another point of view there are many simple techniques that have been used throughout the history of Chinese medicine which require minimal training for one to be able to put them to good use.

An outstanding example of this from Chinese history is referred to as the "Mǎ Dān Yáng 12 heavenly star points." Mǎ Dān Yáng was a famous doctor who formulated a selection of 12 acupuncture points—relatively easy to locate and treat—which an able person could learn to use effectively for treating minor health problems amongst family members or neighbors. In a similar fashion, a trained health-care provider could stock a variety of patent medicines, learn to apply them in a safe way, and be of help to many patients. Or, for example, a competent psychology specialist could quickly learn to recognize TCM patterns—so as to understand in general terms which medicine is most suited for which type of patient, and when to call on an expert for help—and thereby be able to select and administer three or four patent medicines that promote good sleep. This could help patients sleep well—with no side effects—and thus enhance other treatments.

A NOTE REGARDING CONTENT

When the authors wrote this book it was to share their clinical specialization with their peers. The most important themes from their perspective were the ways that TCM addressed schizophrenia and other mental diseases, and the best ways to use it in those regards. Hence the authors discussed not only schizophrenia, but also the treatment of all mental diseases with Chinese medicine. Moreover, they discussed the use of medicinal agents, other ancillary modalities of TCM, and the combined use of TCM treatments with modern medical treatments in the field of mental diseases. They assembled information not only from their own clinical experience, but as well from Chinese medical case studies. This presents one of three important issues that the reader should bear in mind when reading this book.

THE LANGUAGE OF THE MEDICINE

In medical case studies from China, patients with severe mental symptoms are frequently referred to as "schizophrenic." However, there is no such state as schizophrenia in Chinese traditional medicine—recall that a TCM diagnosis is based on the pulse reading and tongue diagnosis, as well as observable and reported symptoms. Thus the patterns of TCM when applied to mental diseases are perceived as varying shades of withdrawal (*diān*) and of mania (*kuǎng*). Whether the patient is or is not schizophrenic according to a Western diagnosis really makes very little difference to what the TCM treatment should be.

The reason the authors explicate schizophrenia at such length is because they want their book to seem modern, up-to-date, and Western. The reason they nonetheless describe treatments in terms of *diān* and *kuǎng* is because that is TCM—that is what they know and that is what works.[1]

---

[1] Readers who would wish to know more about these issues should watch the Paradigm Publications website (www.paradigm-pubs.com). In the early part of 2000 Paradigm will be posting translations of over 20 case studies in which acupuncture was used to treat mental diseases. Besides being useful for showing what acupuncture can do, the case histories also give a certain profile of mental health patients in China, provide a perspective on how TCM is perceived vis-à-vis Western medicine, and sometimes even have entertaining story lines. In sum, they illuminate many cultural issues while demonstrating TCM at its best.

THE PATTERNING OF DISEASE

A second issue for the Western-trained reader may be the impression that the mental diseases which the authors address, particularly in the case studies that are cited, are not prevalently manifested in Western culture, and that therefore the treatments may not be practicable. They may decide that although the treatments explicated can remarkably redress some serious psychological problems, these are not precisely the problems that Westerners are likely to confront either personally or clinically.

While it is true that the social backdrop of disease of all natures in China is significantly different from that in modernized countries, in theory, a good practitioner of TCM is able to accurately determine the underlying pattern of imbalance unique to each patient. Thus, while the specific clinical cases explained might not seem entirely pertinent in a cultural sense, it is important to recognize that it is the modality itself which allows the practitioner to adjust treatment to match their own clinical realities.

THE IDEOLOGICAL PERSPECTIVES OF AN ERA

The authors address some intellectual matters in ways that are sociologically telling. At the time of the authors' original writing, they and their peers held a modernist perspective, and did not consider traditional medicine on a par with Western medicine. Their fundamental belief was that modern medicine would eventually hold the real, scientifically based answers to the serious question of curing illnesses. At the same time, their exposure to Western medicine was limited by cultural and ideological restraints, and thus their understanding of allopathy was somewhat simplistic (though no more than our commensurate understanding of Chinese medicine).

The use of statistics in some cases also seems to reflect the writers' times. While the treatments explained herein do have strong merits, the statistical numbers cited to support the authors' claims can seem unbelievably high—if the treatments were as effective as some of the statistics suggest, all the asylums in China would have been emptied long ago. That has by no means happened. While today the science of biostatistics is becoming more fully integrated in Chinese medical research, against the background of emergence from China's Maoist years these inflated statistics probably reflect nothing more than conformity to the accepted standards and expectations for doctors in China in that era.

A NOTE ABOUT TERMINOLOGY

As someone who could read Chinese comfortably before starting to study TCM, there are several ideas that I would like to share about the value of following the translation protocol developed by Nigel Wiseman, *et al.,* in works like *Glossary of Chinese Medicine* and *A Practical Dictionary of Chinese Medicine.*

Those who do not agree that we should use a shared terminology for translating literature on TCM probably cannot read the original Chinese texts. For those who cannot read the original Chinese, it is hard to explain how repetitively technical terms are used in Chinese TCM literature. We all know that the *Internal Canon* was cited and recited throughout history—in fact, the same terminology has been used over and over, and has simply been applied in different ways in response to historical developments.

As I worked on translating *Soothing the Troubled Mind,* I felt it would be terribly confusing to readers if I did not find some way to make my use of terminology consistent within the text. (Is there any need to mention how difficult it would have been to make it consistent with the work of 10 or 100 other translators?) It was not until I had completed a couple of rough drafts that I heard of Wiseman's approach, and made contact with Bob Felt of Paradigm Publications. I explained my task. He was very interested and sent me a copy of Wiseman's *Glossary of Chinese Medicine.*

It is important for non-Chinese speaking TCM practitioners to understand how easy it was to use the Wiseman terminology to edit my rough draft and make a consistent, worthy translation. With the *Glossary of Chinese Medicine* at hand, I could usually determine which Chinese characters had specific meanings in TCM, and could look them up with ease.

Thus, while I feel that the basic information in *Soothing the Troubled Mind* has many useful aspects, the fact that it ascribes to this shared translation protocol enhances its value many times over. In fact, reading this book may be valuable for no other reason than familiarization with all the terminology in TCM that relates to mental illness. It provides any practitioner of TCM a much clearer understanding of other translational works regarding TCM and mental diseases.

Nevertheless, there are still enhancements to be made to Wiseman's translation protocol. It is not possible that all the words used will ever be perfectly accurate to convey all the original meanings, and the passing of years will undoubtedly continue to extend many parts of the protocol. Thus, there is much to be gained by exploring words that translate uncomfortably, discussing them openly, and deciding the best way to bridge the language barrier.

For example, the two terms that are most frequently used in *Soothing the Troubled Mind* are "mania" and "withdrawal." No one disagrees with the translation of the former; its meaning in English is exactly what it is in Chinese. But "withdrawal" is not a very widespread choice. This is worth exploring given the current state of knowledge transmission.

Many diseases in TCM are discussed in terms of categories with yin and yang aspects. In TCM literature, the two characters *diān* (withdrawal) and *kuǎng* (mania) are used in a combination that means "all mental diseases." If the yang aspect of mental diseases is what we call "mania" in English, what should we call the yin aspect of these disorders?

Some people think the answer is to call it "depression." But the classical definition of depression has certain yang aspects to it, such as the anger that is involved from time to time; so "depression" would be very misleading. Also, "manic depressive" (now more frequently called "bipolar disorder") is a specific diagnosis in psychology. Thus using "depression" as a terminological choice for the translation of *diān* would create further confusion as to its use and meaning in Chinese.

One downside of selecting "withdrawal" is that it is also used in English to describe a stage of substance-abuse recovery. However, if we recognize that it has the clinical meaning of social/emotional/intellectual detachment from reality, we are hard-put to find any other word in English that as aptly summarizes the yin aspects of mental diseases in general.

The final point that I would like to make about Wiseman's translation protocol is that the more we use it, individually and collectively, the more useful it is. There is a vast body of literature available in Chinese that uses a fairly limited technical terminology. When we all agree on how we are going to translate it and speak about it, we will all be able to learn it faster and understand it more clearly. This is a good goal for us to work toward collectively.

AUTHORS' PREFACE

MENTAL DISORDERS, especially schizophrenia, present a serious danger to a healthy society. The rates of mental diseases are quite high in some foreign countries. In France, for example, the rate of drug consumption for mental disorders increased 47% in the last ten years. Consequently, clinical doctors and medical research specialists both domestically and abroad have placed broad emphasis on preventing and treating mental illnesses. After ranking cancer and cardiovascular diseases as first and second priorities, the British medical research committee's five-year plan for 1986-1990 made research into mental disorders the next highest priority.

The authors have practiced acupuncture for many years, and have accumulated valuable experience specifically in treating mental disorders. They feel deeply that acupuncture should be regarded as an effective method for treating mental disorders. Because compiling this book was only intended to cast a brick that would elicit jade, we request cohorts to make criticisms and corrections.

In this book several sections and chapters were researched in the reference resources of Chén Jiā Yáng, Cáo Xī Liàng, Zhāng Féng Chūn, Qín Dé Píng, Zhāng Míng Jiǔ, and others. Please excuse us for not mentioning our gratitude to each individually; we here express our sincere thanks to all.

The Authors

Hang Zhou, September 1987

~ CHAPTER ONE ~
INTRODUCTION

S CHIZOPHRENIA IS A COMMON MENTAL DISORDER afflicting 60-80% of institutionalized mental patients. The symptoms of this disorder are manifold and varied, but the most important characteristics are abnormal intellectual, emotional, and behavioral responses to the surrounding environment. The pathology of this disorder is not yet clearly understood, but hereditary and environmental factors are considered to have an important bearing. Acupuncture and moxibustion produce consistently fine therapeutic results for schizophrenia and other psychological disorders.

China's traditional medicine regards schizophrenia within the context of withdrawal-mania (*diān-kuáng*), and considers it to develop from disharmony of qi and blood with phlegm and fire harassing the upper body. *Líng Shū*, "*Diān Kuáng*" says:

> *When mania (kuáng) arises, [the patient takes] scant rest and [has] no hunger. There are self-delusions of superiority and virtuousness, of discernment and wisdom, and of honor and venerability. [Such patients are] given to cursing day and night.*[1]

---

[1]Translator's note—This identical quotation appears again in Chapter 5, along with the author's explanation in modern Chinese of the classical Chinese that is used in the *Líng Shū*.

Also, *Yī Xué Rù Mén* by Lǐ Chān in the Ming Dynasty states:

> *Mania patients are ferociously mad. In mild cases they act self-important and self-righteous, they like to sing and like to dance; in more serious cases [patients] throw off their clothes and run amok, climb walls and mount the roof. In even more serious cases [patients may] beat their head [against a wall] and scream, be negligent around fire and water, or can have inclinations to murder. This naturally results from inordinate exuberance of the heart fire, superabundance of yang qi, the spirit failing to keep to its abode, and phlegm-fire congestion and exuberance. The crux of treating mania is to descend phlegm and downbear fire.*

This fully describes mania patients and their peculiar features of excitability, high emotions, vocal and physical excesses, and the obviously self-aggrandizing nature of their thoughts.

Qiān Jīn Yào Fāng by Sūn Sī Miǎo in the Tang Dynasty states:

> *When wind enters the yin channels there is withdrawal (diān). The forms can have many extremes. [Some patients] are taciturn and make no sound, [while others] say many things in effusive speeches. They also may sing or cry, moan or laugh. [They may] also sleep or sit in ditches, eat feces and filth, show their naked bodies [in public], rove around all day and night, and ceaselessly curse and cuss.*

Also, *Yī Xué Rù Mén* states:

> *Withdrawal patients are frequently strange. Normally they can speak, but in withdrawal they are deeply taciturn; or if on normal days they do not speak, in withdrawal there is moaning and groaning. ... Often their hearts are not happy.*

This describes withdrawal patients and their high degree of restraint, downcast emotions, reduced vocal and physical actions—even to the point of not talking or moving—and the cognitive sluggishness of their thoughts.

Patients with schizophrenia often have symptoms of both mania (*kuáng*) and withdrawal (*diān*) diseases. They may have the withdrawal tendencies to feeble will, poor self-motivation, unsociability, deep taciturnity, dulled emotional responses, lack of concern about their surroundings, and apathy regarding their appearance. If pushed they do not move and if addressed they do not respond; such is their stuporous condition. It is as if they were stiff like wood. They can also have manic behavior such as excited movements, incoherent speech, explosive behavior, or sudden outbursts where they wreak destruction and injure people.

Ancient scholars recognized the causes of schizophrenia to be of three types. These are: invasions by the six environmental excesses (factors from the natural climate), over-stimulation of the seven affects (mental factors), and other factors (such as fatigue, diet, herbs and medicinal minerals, and accidental injuries). Therefore they say for this disorder, "A thousand forms of suffering do not exceed three types."[2]

Where the *Inner Canon* discusses how each factor from the world of nature can lead to human illness, it says:

If wind, rain, cold, and heat do not encounter vacuity [in a person], an evil is unable to independently do damage.

Regarding the relation between emotional changes and vacuity and repletion in the five viscera, it points out that "when the heart qi is in vacuity there is sorrow; when in repletion there is unceasing laughter." This clearly implies that whether illness results either from factors of the natural environment, or influences from emotional fluctuations, it is dependent on the circumstances of the individual's internal health.

In addition, the ancients took congenital factors into consideration. In *Líng Shū*, "*Yīn Yáng Èr Shí Wǔ Rén*," there is an explanation of different physique types and how each relates to the development of disease.

The three types of factors that cause this disorder are explained as follows.

---

[2]Translator's note—Readers who are not familiar with Chinese medicine may find it useful to know that these three causes are cited as the causes of all diseases, not just schizophrenia. Traditional Chinese doctors try to trace the causes of a patient's disease from these three choices as a step in determining the disease pattern. Thus, even though doctors in ancient times could not have recognized the modern term we use, they would nonetheless have understood it in terms of these three possible origins.

I. INVASIONS OF THE SIX ENVIRONMENTAL EXCESSES

Discussions of the six environmental excesses began in the Spring and Autumn Period. *Zuǒ Zhuàn* records that the physician named Zhào Mèng said:

> With yin environmental excess there is a cold disease; with yang environmental excess there is a hot disease. With wind environmental excess there is disease in the extremities; with rain environmental excess there is abdominal disease. With brightness environmental excess there is disease of the heart; with environmental excess of dark there is disease of confusion.

The phrases "disease in the heart" and "disease of confusion" refer to mental functions. There are numerous historical records of the externally contracted six environmental excesses resulting in delirium, insanity, and other mental disorders. *Elementary Questions,* "*Shēng Qì Tōng Tiān Lún*" states:

> When due to cold, [the disease] is like a turning pivot; [the patient] is frightened in daily life, and spirit qi floats [astray]. When due to summerheat sweating, there is vexation and noisy panting which when stilled gives way to garrulousness.

Zhū Bìng Yuán Hòu Lún states:

> In mania patients, the disease is from wind evil entering a yang [position].

Qiān Jīn Yào Fāng also points out:

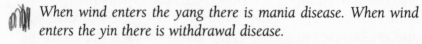

> When wind enters the yang there is mania disease. When wind enters the yin there is withdrawal disease.

The quotations above clearly state that external contractions of the six environmental excesses can be causes of mental disorders.

II. DAMAGE FROM INTEMPERANCE OF THE SEVEN AFFECTS

The seven affects (joy, anger, anxiety, thought, sorrow, fear, and fright) are the basis of typical human mental functions. However, if a certain limit is exceeded and ordinary controls are lost, their influence can lead to disease. Physicians in ancient times gave close attention to these factors for their role in causing psychological abnormalities. For example, *Líng Shū*, "*Diān-Kuáng*" states:

> Mania patients eat ravenously, have tendencies to laugh, but do not show it outwardly. They get [these symptoms] from an occasion of great joy.
>
> Patients with raving speech, fear, tendencies to laugh, and fondness for singing, or ceaseless mad talk, get [these symptoms] from a great fright.

In addition, *Líng Shū*, "*Běn Shén*" says:

> When the heart has apprehensive thought, then the spirit is damaged. When the spirit is damaged then there is uncontrollable fear and dread.
>
> When the spleen has unresolved anxiety, the reflection (stored by the spleen) is damaged. When reflection is damaged then there is chaos.
>
> As to the liver, when sorrow touches one to the core, then the ethereal soul (stored by the liver) is damaged. When the ethereal soul is damaged, there is mania.
>
> As to the lung, when joy and happiness reach their extremes, the corporeal soul (stored by the lung) is damaged. When the corporeal soul is damaged, there is mania.
>
> As to the kidney, when anger abounds unabated, then the memory [zhì—stored by the kidney] is damaged. With a damaged memory, the patient is inclined to forget what he has said.

The *Inner Canon* points out that the five viscera are damaged by their corresponding emotions when the latter become excessive, and posits the view that emotions can overcome each other. For example, *Elementary Questions*, "*Yīn Yáng Yìng Xiàng Dà Lùn*" contains these statements:

> Anger damages the liver; sorrow overcomes anger.
>
> Joy damages the heart; anxiety overcomes joy.
>
> Thought damages the spleen; anger overcomes thought.
>
> Anxiety damages the lung; joy overcomes anxiety.
>
> Fear damages the kidney; thought overcomes fear.

Regarding "visceral agitation in women" and "running piglet disease," *Jīn Guì Yào Luè*, written by Zhāng Zhòng Jīng in the Han Dynasty, says: "These are caught from having fright or fear."

Yī Xué Zhèng Zhuàn by Yú Tuán of the Ming Dynasty states:

[Mania-withdrawal diseases] are mostly in people who have lofty aims that are not attained.

Zhèng Zhì Yào Jué by Dài Sī Gōng of the Ming Dynasty says:

Mania-withdrawal diseases are from depressions of the seven affects.

Yī Xué Rù Mén by Lǐ Chān of the Ming Dynasty says:

People who have unfulfilled plans, who get depressed because they have not accomplished their will, often get this disease.

Zhèng Zhì Zhǔn Shéng by Wáng Kěn Táng, also of the Ming Dynasty, states:

[Withdrawal disease occurs] most often in patients with high ambitions, who do not accomplish what they want.

Jǐng Yuè's Complete Works, by Zhāng Jīng Yuè of the Ming Dynasty, suggested:

Whenever one has no evident disease, but when there is depression, unfulfillment, apprehensive thoughts, or doubts, fright, and fear; these can gradually develop into feeble-mindedness.

Zá Bìng Yuán Liú Xī Zhú by Shěn Jīn Áo of the Qing Dynasty also says:

Occasions of great fear or great joy, great anxiety or great fright, can lead to suffering a loss of [normal] spirit.

The statements above all consider mental factors to be causes of mania and withdrawal diseases.

III. OTHER FACTORS

Yet another explanation is inherited fetal disease. *Elementary Questions* comments:

If born with the disease of madness ... the disease is called a fetal disease. It is contracted while in the mother's womb, and the mother had a certain fright.

Schizophrenia is attributable to the seven affects and the six environmental excesses damaging the viscera and bowels and channels and network vessels. This results in the human body losing regulation of yin and yang, which then creates mental chaos. In particular there may be a series of pathological developments involving qi, blood, phlegm, and fire.

1. QI AND BLOOD

The ancients held that "the hundred diseases arise out of qi." Of the various influences, emotional changes were seen as having an especially important influence on qi. Thus *Elementary Questions,* "Zhū Tòng Lùn" says:

> *I know what it means that the hundred diseases arise out of qi. When there is anger, the qi ascends. When there is joy, the qi slackens. With sorrow the qi disperses. With fear the qi descends. With cold the qi contracts. With heat the qi is discharged. With fright the qi goes into chaos. With taxation the qi is weak. With thought the qi binds.*

In addition, the ancients held the opinion that as "with fright the qi goes into chaos," there may be the abnormal mental occurrence of "the spirit has no place to return to, and cogitation has no place to settle." Moreover, the qi dynamic in disharmony can initiate irregular visceral and bowel functions, and produce all manner of mental symptoms.

Regarding the relation of mental symptoms and the blood, *Elementary Questions,* "Tiáo Jīng Lùn" pointed out:

> *When blood is superabundant there is anger, when insufficient there is apprehension. ...*

> *When blood gathers in the upper body and qi gathers in the lower body, there is vexation, oppression, and irascibility (tendency to anger). When blood gathers in the lower body and qi gathers in the upper body, there is derangement and forgetfulness.*

This is sufficient for us to see that disharmony of qi and blood can initiate mental confusion. In later times, from this foundation, it was thought that blood vacuity and blood stasis could induce mental abnormalities. *Yī Xué Zhèng Zhuàn* by Yú Tuán of the Ming Dynasty points out that "withdrawal [is induced by] insufficiency of heart blood."

Lǐ Chān also had the opinion that withdrawal was from "yin vacuity and scant blood." He pointed out that qi and blood vacuity can be complicated by exuberant, congesting phlegm-fire; the resulting loss of normal heart spirit creates visual and auditory hallucinations, along with symptoms such as nonsensical garbled speech. [He also] refuted the superstition–theory that schizophrenia is from "the work of evil ghosts and demons." [He states,] for example:

> When a patient sees, hears, speaks, and acts absurdly, it is said to be due to the activity of evil spirits. This is just qi and blood in extreme vacuity, the spirit and will in insufficiency, or else it is complicated by phlegm-fire obstructing and predominating, so that the spirit is confused and unsettled. It is not really the work of ghosts and demons.

Regarding blood stasis resulting in illness, *Yī Xué Xīn Wù* by Chén Zhōng Líng of the Qing Dynasty said:

> If a mania patient conforms to the blood stasis type ... blood amasses in the lower burner, and there is uncontrolled urination.

Yī Lín Gǎi Cào by Wáng Qīng Rèn in the Qing Dynasty said:

> In mania-withdrawal, the qi and blood congeal and stagnate, the qi of the brain does not contact with the visceral and bowel qi, and it is the same as if having a dream.

2. PHLEGM AND FIRE

The *Inner Canon* was the earliest source to point out that mania symptoms are initiated by fire, stating: "Excessive agitation and mania are ascribed to fire." Fire and heat are inseparable. Thus, as the *Inner Canon* states:

When an evil is visiting it is heat. When heat is extreme there is aversion to fire. ... When the disease is extreme [the patient] removes his clothes and goes about.

In the Jin Dynasty, Liú Yuán Sù developed the idea that "excessive agitation and mania are ascribed to fire." He particularly emphasized that fire and heat initiate mania:

If presently a patient has yang in exuberance and yin in vacuity, then water is weak and fire is strong. Restrained metal is unable to calm wood, and [the patient] has tendencies to abuse friends. They curse and do not alter their [strange behavior] for either family or strangers.³ They are fond of laughing, have hate and anger, and are manic. This is engendered at root by fire and heat.

We should attribute two Jin-Yuan era physicians, Zhāng Cóng Zhēng and Zhū Dān Xī, with pointing out that phlegm is a factor in epilepsy and mania pathogenesis. *Rú Mén Shì Qīn* by Zhāng Cóng Zhēng states:

[When the liver] constantly plans, and the gallbladder is constantly indecisive, by being bent over without stretching, and holding anger that is not discharged, the heart blood grows dryer by the day. Spleen humor does not move, and phlegm then confounds the orifices of the heart, forming heart wind.

Dān Xī Xīn Fǎ says:

Withdrawal ascribes to yin. Mania ascribes to yang. Withdrawal patients have overabundant joy, and mania patients have overabundant anger ... largely resulting from phlegm binding in the heart and chest.

In this circumstance, the "phlegm" in "phlegm confounding the orifices of the heart" is from chronic mental factors. When the human body's "heart blood grows dryer by the day, and spleen humor is not moving," the result is failure of splenic movement; the conversion of essence forms phlegm, which causes mental

---

³Translator's note—*Bù bì qīn shū* ("do not alter their [strange behavior] for either family or strangers") is a regularly seen phrase in Chinese medical literature. It describes people who are in a mental state such that they behave oddly, and noticeably inappropriately; they do not hide their strange behavior, nor do they discriminate in the way they treat people who would normally be considered socially close or distant to them.

disorders. Phlegm and fire are also closely related, and interact in their effects. As Yú Tuán pointed out, "Mania is from phlegm-fire in repletion and exuberance." *Lèi Zhèng Zhì Cái* by Lín Pèi Qín said:

> *Withdrawal and mania are both from the heart fire itself burning, and phlegm confounding the orifices and network vessels. Thus, at the onset of withdrawal there is a loss of regular emotions, and the form is similar to mania. After a long period of mania the spirit has confusion and blurred vision, and the form is similar to some types of withdrawal.*

These quotations all expound how phlegm and fire cause mental symptoms at various stages of pathological development.

Phlegm and qi are also closely linked. Zhāng Jǐng Yuè pointed out:

> *Withdrawal often arises from phlegm. Whenever qi has some counterflow, and phlegm has some stagnation, they can congest channels and network vessels, and block the orifices of the heart.*

Moreover, Chén Shì Duó held that in treatment of phlegm one must supplement qi:

> *If one indiscriminately treats just phlegm without supplementing qi, sudden death will be unavoidable.*

It can be seen that phlegm confounding the heart orifices has close relations to qi counterflow and qi stagnation, as well as qi vacuity.

In summary of the above explanations, qi, blood, phlegm, and fire are the interrelated constituents of mania-withdrawal pathology. During the Qing Dynasty, Shěn Jīn Áo made advances in synthesizing and explaining all the above theories. He not only covered mania-withdrawal, he also broadly covered fright, palpitations, and fear patterns. In *Zá Bìng Yuán Liú Xī Zhú*, "*Diān-Kuáng Lùn*," he says:

> *Mania-withdrawal is a disease of the heart and of the liver and stomach, inevitably complicated by phlegm and complicated by fire. Withdrawal is due to heart qi vacuity with heat. Mania is due to evil heat in the domain of the heart. These are the causes of*

withdrawal and mania. Withdrawal is ascribed to the bowels and phlegm in the connecting vessels. Therefore it comes and goes. Mania is ascribed to the viscera and it gathers at the heart-governor. Therefore, attacks are unrelenting. These are the causes that lead to both withdrawal and mania.

Shěn Jīn Áo also said:

The cause of withdrawal is losing will for plans and hopes, and is formed from unremitting depression. The cause of mania is repressed yang qi that cannot be coursed beyond. Moreover, the heart spirit must be consumed and dissipated such that with qi vacuity it is unable to prevail. Thus, when phlegm and fire madly invade the upper body they result in two diseases. Thus, the origins of withdrawal and mania are the same.

Modern medical science regards schizophrenia as a disorder that is still not fully understood. According to reviews of current research articles, however, it is explained as the result of many causes. Textbooks in China summarize these influences in four aspects: heredity, premorbid personality traits, environment, and physical health. Mayer-Gross *et al.* consider such influences to include heredity, constitution, and the endocrine, metabolic, and central nervous systems, as well as precipitating factors which may be illnesses or psychological factors. The Japanese journal *Seishin Yihaku (Psychological Medical Sciences)* summarizes the roots of this illness in two types: hereditary and psychological. There are also those who summarize the two types as hereditary and environmental.

In fact, any biological phenotype, no matter whether it is physiological or pathological, must fundamentally be the combined result of hereditary and environmental factors; it is only that the relative strengths of the two factors vary. The pathological causes of schizophrenia are no exception to this rule. Therefore we should not incline toward favoring one of the two, but it should be understood that the two have complimentary effects. Heredity is the internal cause of illness, while environment is the external cause of illness. The external cause acts via the internal cause to stimulate an effect.

Moreover, the internal and external factors are mutually convertible. Sometimes it is difficult to determine what is caused by heredity, and what is caused by the environment. If a child's personality type is similar to his mother's, perhaps this is due in part to heredity and in part to environmental post-natal influences. Schizophrenia develops when environmental influences trigger congenital tendencies. It occurs when someone who has these tendencies meets a relatively great environmental pressure that surpasses the endurance of the nervous system, or if the internal environment is disturbed.

A study was conducted by scholars in China on a group of 100 schizophrenia patients, with a control group of 100 normal individuals. Using SYS-8 computerized multiple regression analysis, they analyzed 22 types of causes for onset of this disorder. This analysis indicates that five types of factors are closely associated with the onset of schizophrenia. They are:

~ Poor intrapersonal relations during childhood
~ History of family heredity
~ Tense family atmosphere during childhood
~ Evident introversion tendencies before onset
~ Some unpleasant occurrence during gestation or parturition.

Based on our clinical experience, schizophrenia patients have all been exposed to marked mental stimuli before onset, and such stimuli are a crucial circumstance for the disorder to manifest. The strength of the stimulus, and whether it is sufficient to elicit an episode, depends on the patient's particular constitution and his state of health at that time. In certain people a very slight, insignificant cause can trigger the onset of psychosis.

Others can receive a great stimulus, yet withstand it very calmly. For example, during World War I and World War II, in the abominable conditions of wrecked families and ruined lives, there simply was no clear increase in the number of schizophrenic patients. Many reports argue that this indicates hereditary elements are responsible, but in clinical practice these claims are only useful as reference. At the present there are no completely clear explanations of the pathogenesis for schizophrenia.

Schizophrenia has the following three attributes:

1. Before onset there are often personality characteristics of eccentricity, hesitancy, and stubbornness, which are identifiable as characteristics of a schizophrenic personality.

2. Frequently onset occurs during adolescence or early adulthood; it may arise slowly or quickly, but usually onset is due to mental trauma.

3. A very slight minority of patients can recover on their own, while a portion of the patients can be cured. However, the majority of patients have recurrent episodes of the disorder, in a gradually worsening progression.

Schizophrenia patients can be divided according to clinical symptoms as follows:

1. Simple type. This type usually occurs in adolescence with an indistinct onset. At onset the condition is not apparent, but it gradually develops to a loss of normal mentality.

2. Hebephrenic type. This type occurs during adolescence with a relatively rapid onset of disease. The symptoms, which are very pronounced, include hallucinations, delusions, and excited, impulsive behavior.

3. Catatonic type. The onset of this type of disorder is also sudden. Signs include a stuporous state, waxy flexibility, mechanical movements, or pigheadedness and stubbornness.

4. Paranoid type. This is also called the delusive type. Onset is gradual, patients are relatively older, and delusions are the major symptom. It can be accompanied by symptoms such as hallucinations and abnormal or eccentric behavior. In severe cases, there may be impulsive behavior. Patients may injure people or wreak destruction; some are unable to manage their own lives, and frequently they require protection or admission to a mental hospital for treatment.

There are numerous records of acupuncture treatments for mania-withdrawal in Chinese medical books throughout history. There are also many orally transmitted special needling methods that still exist today. In 1951 there were reports of Mr. Zhū Liǎn using acupuncture to treat schizophrenia. This attracted the attention of the medical community and [was influential] in furthering the widespread use of acupuncture in this field.

According to incomplete statistics, in the last 30 years more than 200 articles have provided reports and data in this regard.

In the 1960's the outstanding contribution of acupuncture to the treatment of mental disorders was electroacupuncture shock therapy. The method of insulin shock therapy for mental disorders requires large quantities of medicine, and a long treatment course; it also incurs complications and side effects. Electroacupuncture shock therapy is thus superior to the insulin method.

Deep needling on GV-16 *(fēng fǔ)* for the paranoid types and hebephrenic types has a good therapeutic effect; when combined with pharmaceutical sedatives, the effectiveness rate reached 98.7%, which is 30-40% higher than solely using drugs. The shortcoming of this method is that mastering the manipulation technique is difficult, and with mistaken punctures serious accidents can occur.[4]

There are reports of using vessel-pricking therapy [in the treatment of mental disorders]. For example, pricking small blood veins at locations such as *tài yáng* (Greater Yang, M-HN-9), *wěi zhōng* (BL-40), *qū chí* (LI-11), and *fēng lóng* (ST-40), and letting a few drops of blood out has had a success rate as high as 70% in treatment of mania patients of the heat-repletion type.

There are also reports of catgut [suture-]embedding therapy for treatment of schizophrenia. In such treatments #0 catgut, 1.5cm long, is implanted at *yǎ mén* (GV-15), *dà zhuī* (GV-14), *táo dào* (GV-13), and in the area of the ear. Each time 2-4 points are selected, and treatments are performed once or twice per week. Ten treatments comprise one course. The effectiveness rate reached 94.1%.

In addition, acupuncture point injection therapy with small doses also accomplished distinctive effectiveness rates. Researchers

---

[4]Translator's note—The point in question is located directly below the external occipital protuberance. Some acupuncturists claim almost miraculous results when needling these points; other acupuncturists contend that the dangers are too great. See p. 108 for a fuller discussion of this point and the concerns surrounding it.

injected less than 16 units of insulin per patient on a daily basis to treat 509 cases of schizophrenia, with an effectiveness rate of 92.3%. Of these, 70.5% had outstanding improvements. There were also others who used small dosages of substances such as chlorpromazine, tardan, tangkuei *(dāng guī)* injection, or placenta tissue fluid and they also noted encouraging results.

~ CHAPTER TWO ~
CLINICAL SYMPTOMATOLOGY
AND CLASSIFICATIONS

THE CLINICAL SYMPTOMS of schizophrenia are from all perspectives quite complex. Not only do the manifestations vary from one patient to another, they can vary in individual patients during different periods. Some patients have continuous atypical mental symptoms after onset of the disorder, while others have recurrent acute episodes.

In cases where the disorder develops slowly, people generally are unable to recognize it as such. They may understand it to be a personality problem or a problem in thinking. The great majority of patients exhibit an attitudinal problem. They do not recognize disease in themselves and are incapable of taking initiative to seek medical help, which results in regrettable delays.

I. CLINICAL SYMPTOMATOLOGY

The following is an introduction to the commonly seen symptoms of schizophrenia.

1. THOUGHT DISORDERS

Thought disorders are a defining feature of schizophrenia. The term "thought disorders" refers to unfocused thinking, or thinking that is divorced from reality, and lacking an objective, practical nature. This manifests in incoherent speech in which statements do not build on each other; there is confusion, incomplete thoughts, and lack of order. Between sentences there is a lack of relation internally or in meaning. Sometimes a patient will suddenly stop speaking, or while speaking on one theme will suddenly interject a completely unrelated sentence. At other times patients use neologisms that a normal person cannot comprehend.

Some patients have disordered speech that is totally lacking in a central theme or any real meaning. Other patients will have acute episodes where they yell the whole day without ceasing, or talk aloud to themselves in incoherent, incomplete sentences. There are also patients who remain completely silent, and do not respond to even the most persistent inquiry.

This form of thought disorder is also apparent in the letters and other writings of these patients, which are mostly muddled and incomprehensible to others.

2. EMOTIONAL DISORDERS

Patients may develop emotional apathy at an early stage. Toward their families they are distant, cold, or even antagonistic. Their emotional responses are dulled, and they show a lack of concern for their surroundings. Frequently the whole day can be spent sitting at home in boredom, with apparently no inner feelings about either happy or sad events; when they do respond, their facial expressions are dull and lifeless.

Some patients have emotional changes with many extremes. Joy, anger, grief, and happiness interchange so quickly that it mystifies anyone trying to comprehend the causes. Some patients have inappropriate affects. For example, they may carelessly narrate the most painful event of their life, or shed tears over a subject that would make most people happy.

3. DISORDERS OF VOLITION

Disorders of volition are explained as activities of the will that are reduced or lacking. The manifestations are reduced strength to move, reduced initiative and enthusiasm, and behavior that is lazy and listless. They do not aspire to social interaction, work, or studies. Such patients have a slovenly personal appearance and do not maintain their personal hygiene. Some develop contradicting emotions where they think over and over about even the most simple daily encounter until it becomes difficult to resolve. Other patients have stereotyped movements or imitative movements; they mechanically obey or defy and have other symptoms of catatonia.

4. PERCEPTUAL DISORDERS

These are commonly seen symptoms in schizophrenia. Perceptual disorders are the hallucinations and delusions that schizophrenic patients manifest.

A. HALLUCINATIONS

Hallucinations often occur in circumstances when a patient's consciousness is perfectly clear. Among the [range of] hallucinations, auditory hallucinations (especially linguistic auditory hallucinations) are most frequently encountered. Sensory, olfactory, visual, and visceral hallucinations are more rare.

The contents of hallucinations are usually simple and unchanging, and often cause the patient to be unhappy. Patients may hear someone talking to them from out of nowhere, or hear someone command that they do something. These are genuine hallucinations in which the sound is clear to the patient. They may obey the commanding voice, even to carry out dangerous deeds. Such patients may have a dialogue with an hallucinated voice and mutter to themselves, or turn one ear to a listening position, or be transfixed by the hallucinatory experience. Patients may laugh to themselves, or talk and speak to themselves as if surreptitiously commenting.

Visual hallucinations may also occur, such as glimpsing apparitions that are simply not there. Some patients hallucinate putrid smells, the sensations of bugs crawling on them, or feelings of electric current passing through their body.

B. DELUSIONS

The contents of delusions are multifarious and are usually bizarre, sudden, and divorced from reality. Delusions have various manifestations. Some patients feel themselves to be the victim of an adverse conspiracy, and are said to have delusions of persecution. Some have exaggerated conceit; they feel their capabilities, position, and wealth all surpass that of others. These are called delusions of grandeur. Other patients have delusions of self-doubt and blame; these are known as delusions of self-accusation. Some patients are suspicious of others without having the slightest provocation, such as suspecting that their spouse is secretly dating another person, having improper sexual relations, and so forth. This form is termed delusions of jealousy. There is also a kind called "erotic madness,"[1] where the patient feels that someone has fallen in love with them. They will usually pester that person ceaselessly. This is referred to as delusions of deep love. Some patients feel that electricity, ultrasonic waves, or machines control their body, behaviors, and thoughts.

The explanations above cover the basic symptomatic manifestations of schizophrenia. In clinical practice, patients most often have one of these symptoms primarily, but it can also happen that several symptoms occur simultaneously in one patient. For example, frequently a patient who primarily exhibits thought disorders will simultaneously have signs of emotional disorders, such as excited shouting, manic laughter, or grimacing. Some patients who exhibit restrained movement as their predominant manifestation may mutely stand to one side and maintain an exaggerated posture. They may also pose rigidly and neither talk nor move, or else have defiant behavior and not accept food to eat. It is possible that during some periods they will have episodes of being excited and disturbed, wreaking destruction and injuring people; after the episode they return to a stiff posture.

---

[1]Translator's note—The expression *huā diān* means literally "flowery madness." Among its many usages, the word *huā* has connotations of promiscuity.

II. CLINICAL CLASSIFICATIONS

Schizophrenia is commonly divided into several clinical types. These types reflect the specific clinical features of patients in the various stages of disorder development. They are founded on variations in basic conditions, duration of disorder, and prognosis. With long-term observation, one sees that the clinical type each patient manifests possesses a corresponding static nature.

However, some patients have disorders that evolve with clinical developments and transmute from one type to another. Besides these considerations, patients in the early stages of schizophrenia do not necessarily have entirely clear clinical manifestations. After prolonged devolution and deterioration to the later stages of mental decline, the transformations in each type tend toward recalcitrance. Only rarely is there reversion to the original type. The current divisions of schizophrenia are: simple type, hebephrenic type, catatonic type, and paranoid type. Whatever does not conform to these types, or when a case is atypical, it is categorized as an undifferentiated type.

1. SIMPLE-TYPE SCHIZOPHRENIA

If a schizophrenic patient has few or no associated symptoms throughout the course of their disorder, and primarily maintains the basic symptomatology, this is called the simple type of schizophrenia. This type of patient usually has the illness in their younger years. The disorder has a slow onset, develops steadily, and abates by itself only infrequently. The primary clinical manifestations are daily worsening eccentricity, passivity, disinterest in the surroundings, and emotional coldness toward others. In extreme cases patients lack even the slightest feeling for close family members. Such patients are mentally listless, have dulled responses, are loathe to engage in activity, and are careless about maintaining personal hygiene and appearance. Their school grades go down, work capacity declines, and frequently they stare blankly or stupidly, or cover their heads and sleep. These are the basic symptoms of this type. Progressions and developments could manifest various associated symptoms. For example, a patient's speech could show confusion, or have strange, illogical deductions that are incomprehensible. Others manifest all kinds of hallucinations. Some laugh or cry for no reason, behave oddly, or impulsively attack people. There are also patients who neither eat nor drink, nor do they talk or move. They behave as if made of wood.

In the early stages this type of patient can be misdiagnosed as having a problem in thinking or a personality problem. If in the early stages the patient exhibits insomnia, headaches, or mental apathy, they may be diagnosed as having neurasthenia. Frequently several years pass before it is discovered that a serious condition has been developing.

2. HEBEPHRENIC-TYPE SCHIZOPHRENIA

The hebephrenic type of schizophrenia usually occurs during adolescence. The disorder may have an abrupt or gradual onset. When the disorder occurs with abrupt onset, it usually reaches a climax within a short period. We must point out that while patients of this type are mostly in adolescence, it is not true that all youths who develop schizophrenia are necessarily of the hebephrenic type.

The mental activity of a hebephrenic patient is lazy and deranged. They tear things apart, and very often languish in empty thoughts about so-called "science" and "philosophy," idly speculating on the fundamental philosophical issues of human existence. They have an aggrandized appreciation for their own powers of invention and creation, and haphazardly seek to actualize their "grand schemes and great enterprises." This type also has the special characteristic of obvious sexual issues, such as excessive sexual drive, and quite frequently impulsive [sexual] behavior. Schizophrenic patients of the hebephrenic type have irregular emotions of joy and anger; in a moment there can be vast changes. Their behavior is naive, unsophisticated, and frequently controlled by hallucinations and delusions.

3. CATATONIC-TYPE SCHIZOPHRENIA

This type of schizophrenia patient is usually young and the onset of this disorder is quite rapid. Early phase manifestations are low spirits and lack of motivation, reduced appetite, laziness, and reduced physical movements. The patient will have neither interest nor emotional involvement in any issues or concerns. As the disorder progresses, it may differentiate as one of two types: catatonic stupor or catatonic excitement.

A. CATATONIC STUPOR

Patients who manifest catatonic stupor appear emotionally cold, with noticeably reduced speech and activity, such that at times they may hold a standing or sitting pose for several hours without moving. They may have rigid movements, rigid speech, imitative movements, imitative speech, disobedience, or other such symptoms. During periods of severe onset, such patients do not speak, do not move, do not drink, do not eat; both eyes are tightly closed or held in a frozen stare, and there is no facial expression. If pushed, they do not move; if called, they do not answer. They respond to no stimulus whatsoever. Although the bladder and large intestine fill with large quantities of urine and feces, they do not excrete. A large quantity of saliva fills the mouth cavity, but it is neither swallowed nor spit out, and it eventually overflows. Overall body musculature exhibits increased tension, or wax flexibility may arise. Brief occurrences of this condition may last just a few hours; prolonged cases endure for several years and then gradually abate. Some cases may conclude suddenly, and a portion of such patients will then enter a condition of catatonic excitement.

B. CATATONIC EXCITEMENT

Manifestations of catatonic excitement often have abrupt onset. Patients are agitated and excited; their behavior is explosive and they often wreak destruction and injure people. Their hallucinations are commonly rich and profuse. This condition normally lasts a few hours or a few days, and afterwards it abates. Patients may enter a stuporous condition, or manifest continuous stereotyped motions. At severely critical times there may be unceasing agitated motions throughout the day and night that result in fatigue or exhaustion.

4. PARANOID-TYPE SCHIZOPHRENIA

The paranoid type is also called the delusive type, and among the different kinds of schizophrenia is the one most frequently seen. Onset occurs later in life for this type than for the other types, often after the age of thirty. It also arises slowly.

The primary clinical symptom is delusions. At onset, patients are sensitive and have many suspicions. Gradually they develop delusions of reference, or the constant feeling that all phenomena occurring in their purview must refer to them. If someone coughs, it is directed at them; if another person spits, it shows disdain for them; if others are chatting, the discussion is about them. They even suspect that newspaper articles or TV or radio broadcasts all allude to them. As the delusions of reference involve a broader scope, it becomes easier to develop delusions of persecution. This is when the patient becomes convinced that everything surrounding him has been set up by someone in order to harm him.

A patient with such persecution delusions firmly believes that his adversaries will employ any method (including the most advanced electronic apparatus) to injure him; his behavior is under observation, his health is being destroyed, his life is in danger. Clinically, delusions of persecution are the most frequently seen. Beyond this there are hypochondria and delusions of jealousy, self-guilt, and affectation.

The vast majority of patients of this type also have hallucinations, with auditory hallucinations most frequently encountered. Hallucinations and delusions often control the behavior and emotions of such patients. As a result, they may injure people, harm themselves, or have other dangerous behavior.

Those who spontaneously recuperate are rare. In the early stages, character changes in patients are often not apparent. Except at times when patients do not wish to expose the content of their hallucinations or delusions, other aspects of their mental activities undergo no change. Once begun, there is a long period within which the patient can engage in normal working life and easily remain undiagnosed. Generally speaking, disorders of the delusive type mostly develop slowly. However, we should recall that patients can suffer acute bouts of schizophrenia as a result of certain mental stimuli or physically induced causes (such as infection, poisoning, trauma, or exhaustion).

~ CHAPTER THREE ~
DIAGNOSIS AND ESSENTIALS OF
DIFFERENTIAL DIAGNOSIS

DIAGNOSIS OF SCHIZOPHRENIA is primarily based on clinical manifestations. By understanding a patient's case history and performing a psychological examination, one can analyze the illness and formulate conclusions concerning the diagnosis.

I. COMPILING THE MEDICAL HISTORY

Patients with schizophrenia frequently do not admit that they are ill, and will rarely seek medical help on their own initiative. Thus, family, neighbors, friends, workmates, or representatives of their work unit must supply the case history. When a case history is compiled the patient should not be present. To understand the case, inquiry should emphasize determining the course of disease, the home situation, and the personal history. Determining crucial issues—such as what triggered onset of the condition or manifestations of delusions—calls for thorough investigation and verification with detailed record keeping.

II. PSYCHOLOGICAL EXAMINATION

One method for understanding a patient's psychological makeup, thoughts, emotions, and memories, is to observe his behavior and to establish contact with him through conversation. While undertaking the psychological examination, one should meticulously observe a patient's movements and expressions. One should pay attention to whether answers are relevant to questions, and whether or not there are observable signs of decline in mental capacity such as delusions, hallucinations, or poor memory.

Additionally, one should assess the patient's attitude toward his own state. Detailed questioning that probes all aspects of the patient's problems (from the superficial to the deeper levels) provides for a maximum grasp of the patient's mental activity.

When excited and quarrelsome, or taciturn and non-verbal patients are uncooperative during an examination, it is possible that different timing or circumstances may enable one to make helpful observations. Some patients will conceal their symptoms on initial contact with a doctor. They may offer explanations or denials of their case history, and discuss everything clearly and logically. Consequently, some cases require a prolonged period to allow for an accurate diagnosis. Standard physical examination and supplementary laboratory tests are indispensable. The goal of these measures is to rule out misdiagnosis of many disorders (such as brain tumor or certain kinds of poisoning), as long-term research has yet to develop reliable methods of laboratory testing for diagnosing schizophrenia itself.

III. DIFFERENTIAL DIAGNOSIS

When diagnosing schizophrenia, it is most important to differentiate it from the following categories of disorders.

1. MANIC-DEPRESSIVE SYNDROME[1]

Also named affective psychosis, or cyclic psychosis, this is an emotional activity disorder with the basic feature of excessive highs and lows. There are repetitious occurrences that tend to abate naturally without treatment. Looking at the duration of the

---

[1]Translator's note—Subsequent to the time of original publication, the term "bipolar disorders" has come to replace the descriptive "manic-depressive." Here, the author's choice of characters supports the use of the term "manic-depressive."

disorder, the majority of cases abate in three to six months. During periods of cessation, everything is as normal and there is no retention of psychological shortcomings. A minority of patients endure prolonged, uncured disorders that become chronic. There may be episodes of either a manic or a depressive state; it is also possible to have both simultaneously, or interchanging episodes of the two with intervals of cessation, or cyclical attacks.

The states of mania and of depression are opposite emotional disorders. However, observation of the basic nature of each reveals that they are two differing manifestations of the same illness. Manic-depressive syndrome occurs less frequently than schizophrenia, comprising approximately two to three percent of residential patients in mental health institutions.

Schizophrenia can also accompany the condition of manic-depressive syndrome. When a patient simultaneously has thought disorders, eccentric behavior, and relatively many hallucinations, or when their psychomotility is maladjusted, the differential diagnosis is schizophrenia.

2. REACTIVE PSYCHOSIS

Also known as heart-caused (*xīn yīn xìng jīng shén bìng*) psychosis, this disorder results from severe or prolonged psychological factors. The occurrence rate is 1.6–3.1% of residential patients in mental health institutions. Patients usually manifest either of two conditions: psychomotor excitement or psychomotor depression. While the clinical manifestations of this disorder have individual variations, the contents of the clinical psychotic state, as well as psychological elements that cause the disorder, still have close interrelations. This is the defining feature of reactive psychosis. If a patient's mental state departs from this theme and becomes impossible to comprehend, then perhaps it is not the illness at hand but another psychosis.

Mental stimuli can provoke schizophrenia; however, there is the gradual appearance of "schizoid" manifestations; symptoms become increasingly chaotic, and it becomes impossible for ordinary people to comprehend the patient. Then it is not appropriate to retain the diagnosis of reactive psychosis. Reactive psychosis in brief cases may last just a few days; extended cases will abate within a few weeks. A minority of cases continue for up to 2–3 months. The prognosis is usually considered good, but a few patients have sequelae such as insomnia, headaches, easily disturbed emotions, reduced memory, and other conditions of neurosis.

3. NEUROSES

This group of disorders results from temporary loss of adjustment in cerebral functions. The maladjustment is from various mental elements incurring excessive tension in higher nervous activity. The most frequently seen disorders of this type are neurasthenia, hysteria, compulsive neurosis, and many kinds of visceral neurosis (such as cardiovascular neurosis and gastrointestinal neurosis). These are individually explained as follows:

A. NEURASTHENIA

This is a commonly seen type of neurasthenic neurosis. The primary manifestations are exhaustion, nervousness, insomnia, hypochondria, anxiety, and worry. The early stages of schizophrenia can manifest like a condition of neurasthenia. However, a neurasthenia patient will take initiative to get medical help, and will follow the treatment wholeheartedly. A schizophrenia patient, in contrast, has no concern for his state and will not take measures to get medical assistance.

B. HYSTERIA

This disorder mostly occurs in female patients. The clinical manifestations include mental disorders (hysterical emotional attacks) and physical functional impediments (hysterical paralysis, tremors, fainting, and aphonia, or even perceptual disorders and visceral and autonomic nerve disorders). The special clinical traits are thick emotional overtones, exaggerations, susceptibility to suggestion, and episodic attacks with complete normalcy during the intervals. All forms of clinical testing show no positive confirmation.

C. OBSESSIONAL NEUROSIS

This form of neurosis is primarily marked by obsessions. Patients perform repetitive actions which they recognize as inappropriate, but they have no way to free themselves from the related thoughts, emotions, and behavior. Feelings of anxiety and worry are often associated with such actions. They are fully self-aware and normally no behavior occurs that is serious or dangerous.

Schizophrenics may also manifest an obsession, but the contents are absurd and mental stimulation is not a clear factor. Additionally, their self-awareness is lacking; they are emotionally cold and maladjusted, and they have thought disorders, hallucinations, and eccentric behavior. These symptoms are all different from obsessional neurosis.

D. VISCERAL NEUROSIS

The clinical manifestations of this disorder are primarily abnormal functions of visceral organs.[2] Simultaneously there may be insomnia, headaches, amnesia, poor ability to concentrate, anxiety, and other symptoms of a neurotic state. Examination shows that the corresponding organs have no organic changes.

In summary, neurosis and schizophrenia are two completely different kinds of disorders. Causes, pathology, clinical manifestations, and transformations are entirely dissimilar.

4. EPILEPTIC PSYCHOSIS

Epileptic psychosis forms one stage within the general development of epilepsy. It has the usual characteristics of epilepsy with multiple seizures. Before and after the occurrence of mental disorders, or possibly simultaneous to the manifestation of the disorder, there are either grand mal or petit mal seizures. Frequently, the nature of this condition relates to the mental experiences of prodromal epilepsy signs and confusion.

---

[2]Translator's note—Modern Western terminology does not appear to have a clear correspondence to the Chinese classification of "visceral neurosis." However, the descriptive is fairly straightforward.

Epileptic psychosis often occurs after ten or more years of epileptic seizures. At this time seizures are gradually decreasing, and auditory hallucinations and delusions then continue occurring. However, a patient with epileptic psychosis is usually able to remain normal emotionally, and has quite good relations with people. This can differentiate them from schizophrenics who manifest eccentricity, laziness, and emotional incompatibility with others.

5. SYMPTOMATIC PSYCHOSIS

A person's mind and body are a unified whole. Mental disorders can have physical symptoms; diseases of the body can have mental symptoms. When psychotic symptoms are part of the overall clinical symptoms of a somatic disease, it is then called symptomatic psychosis.

Each and every physical illness can cause varying degrees of mental disorders. For the most part they may be categorized as diseases that are either infectious, toxic, or somatic. When somatic diseases cause mental disorders, most mental symptoms improve as the somatic disease declines, so the prognosis is usually good. However, there are some patients who retain mental disorders after the somatic disease has improved, manifesting such symptoms as auditory hallucinations, impeded memory, and thought disorders.

We must point out that although somatic diseases can cause mental abnormalities, not all cases with simultaneous mental abnormalities and somatic diseases are necessarily symptomatic psychosis. Not a few mental patients have somatic diseases that are only provoking factors. As soon as the somatic disease is cured one can then differentiate a clear diagnosis.

6. CLIMACTERIC PSYCHOSIS

This type of psychosis is induced by mental factors or decline of endocrine function during old age. The primary clinical manifestations are feelings of anxiety or worry, and development of certain hallucinations or delusions. There may also be insomnia, headache, poor memory, heart palpitations, or constriction in the chest, and other kinds of neurosis. The age range for female patients is generally between 45 and 55, or just around the time of menopause. Male patients are generally between 50 and 60. Patients are more frequently female than male.

Climacteric psychosis is definitely not the only psychosis that can occur in this age group. Besides occurring at this stage of life, there must also be the specific clinical traits of this psychosis. According to dissimilarities in basic conditions, climacteric psychosis is usually divided into the following three types: climacteric syndrome, primarily with manifestations of neurosis; climacteric depression, primarily with psychotic symptoms of worry, tension, depression, and hypochondria; and climacteric delusion, primarily with delusions accompanied by hallucinations.

7. SENILE PSYCHOSIS

Also called senile dementia, this disorder mostly occurs after the age of 60. It is a form of progressive mental decline that occurs in a body which is undergoing old age. The primary pathology is encephalatrophy. The special clinical feature of this disorder is a slow onset with progressive decline of intellectual capacity and personality traits.

Memory disorders are the most notable development. In serious cases the patients can forget their own name, and lose recognition of their own children. More critical disorders of orientation and comprehension develop gradually, such that in extreme cases, for example, after walking for a few steps they cannot find their way back home. A minority of patients develop psychomotor excitement against the background of dementia, or manifest momentary absurd delusions and hallucinations. Normally the disorder lasts just a few years; frequently patients die of infection or old age.

8. CEREBRAL ARTERIOSCLEROTIC PSYCHOSIS

Also known as arteriosclerotic dementia, this illness is from sclerosis of arteries in the brain influencing the supply of blood to brain tissues and precipitating a mental disorder. The age of most patients is over 50, and patients are slightly more often male than female.

In the early stages, the clinical manifestations of this form are similar to neurasthenia, and the progression of the disorder is slow. Frequently there are fluctuations. There may be long or short intervals of remission. Several years (even over ten years) can pass before there is a transition to arteriosclerotic brain disease.

As a case gradually develops, thought disorders eventually reach the stage of dementia. At this stage, strength of memory, decision-making, comprehension, and thinking are clearly in decline, while creativity and enthusiasm are lost. Nevertheless, the patient is still able to maintain their basic personality for a long period. Because they recognize that they have an illness, this is considered "localized dementia." This is an interesting feature that can be of useful diagnostic significance.

~ CHAPTER FOUR ~
PREVENTION

SCHIZOPHRENIA NOT ONLY CAUSES the utmost suffering to patients and their families, it also affects productivity and social tranquility. Thus, prevention of schizophrenia is clearly important. Medical scholars in our ancient dynasties understood identification of patterns and had a well-developed conception of preventive medicine. *Sù Wèn, "Sì Qì Diào Shén Dà Lún"*[1] says:

> *The sages of antiquity did not treat those who were already sick, but those who were not sick, and did not intervene where unrest had already broken out, but where there was as yet no unrest, then this is what is meant. When a disease has already broken out, and is only then treated with medicaments, or when unrest has broken out and only then does one intervene to impose order, would that not be just as late as to wait for thirst before digging a well or to wait to go into battle before casting weapons?*

Using preventive therapy effectively avoids or reduces the suffering of patients. Moreover, such treatment can enhance the capacity of the central nervous system to function efficiently. Because the causes of schizophrenia are complex and vast, multi-faceted prevention measures are required.

---

[1]Translator's note—The translation of this passage from the *Sù Wèn* has been borrowed from Paul U. Unschuld, in his book, *Chinese Medicine.*

I. CREATING A HEALTHY MENTAL LIFESTYLE

In recent years the theory of "stress" has been employed to investigate the workings of mental illnesses. It is a relatively new direction for research work in pathopsychology and psychiatry. According to Selye's original definition, the basic definition of "stress" is the sum of all the non-specific effects of factors (stressors) which act upon the body.[2]

Stressors are generally divided into two broad types: somatic stressors and psychological stressors. Psychological stressors include a wide variety of psychosocial elements that create a stimulus; these are known as "psychological stimuli" or "mental stimuli."

A study was done that investigated 189 cases of schizophrenia. The analysis showed that over 60% of the patients had distinct psychological stressors preceding the first onset of this illness. While this clearly shows that over half of the cases were related to psychological stress, only $1/7$ to $1/3$ of the cases had distinct psychological stressors preceding subsequent attacks. This means that the majority of cases had a distinct mental stressor before the onset of illness. That source also pointed out that the contents of psychological stressors spread to all aspects of life and society, and their nature and forms tend to multiply; therefore, the contents of psychological stressors have a non-specific nature.

In ancient times, Chinese medical scholars emphasized the role of mental factors in creating illness. They held that fluctuations of the seven affects created damage to the spirits of the five viscera, which then caused mental abnormalities and all manner of disease. Moreover, "qi" was used to summarize illnesses from the seven affects.

---

[2]Translator's note—See Hans Selye, *The Stress of Life* (New York, McGraw-Hill Book Company), p.42, where Selye contends that stress designates the sum of all the non-specific effects of factors (normal activity, disease producers, drugs, etc.) which can act upon the body. He emphasizes that stress is a specific syndrome from non-specific causes.

Qi circulates cyclically and unifies the whole body; it maintains health in the human body; thus it is said:

The spirit desires and seeks wholeness, the qi desires and seeks harmony.

And further:

When there is anger, the qi ascends; when there is joy, the qi slackens; with sorrow the qi disperses; with fear the qi descends; with fright the qi binds.

The hundred diseases are thus generated. Regarding this mechanism it is said:

With anger the qi counterflows; in extreme there is retching of blood, regurgitation, and qi counterflow; thus, the qi ascends. With joy the qi is in harmony and the will outthrusts; construction and defense are free and uninhibited; therefore, the qi slackens. With sorrow the heart tie is tense; the lungs spread and the lobes raise, the two burners do not have free flow, constructive and defensive do not spread, while heat is in the middle; thus, qi disperses. With fear the upper burner blocks; blockage makes the qi return, and returning makes the lower burner distend; therefore, qi does not move. With fright the heart has nothing to rely on, the spirit has no refuge, and thoughts are not stable; therefore, the qi binds.

Obviously, when there is internal damage from emotions, initially it is the *qi* that undergoes a transformation, and the diseases that result are quite varied. Hence Cháo Yuán Fāng of the Sui Dynasty said: "The hundred diseases begin out of qi."

The chaos that ultimately occurs within individual viscera and their functions is the effect of the mental state upon the body's health during the critical period. Thus, as far as nurturing health and preventing diseases, the ancients paid unusually close attention to protecting and nurturing the mind. They thought that "accumulating essence and completely perfecting the spirit are the grand methods for cultivating health." *Líng Shū*, "*Běn Shén*" says:

When the wise cultivate health, they must know appropriate [degrees of] heat and cold through the four seasons; they harmonize joy and anger while staying in a calm home. They moderate yin and yang while adjusting what is hard and soft.

Chinese physicians hold that "to safeguard and nourish the mind" means that the mind should have an appropriate degree of tranquility, and emotions should not suffer undue or excessive fluctuation. The mind should be peaceful, cheerful, and happy. *Sù Wèn*, "*Shàng Gǔ Tiān Zhēn Lùn*" states:

On the outside, do not tax the body with work; on the inside, do not suffer with thinking. Take tranquil pleasures as essential, and accept one's attainments as successes. With the body not worn out and the mind not dissipated, one will possibly age to one hundred.

This simply instructs people to restrain their desires, avoid pursuing overly ambitious delusions, and to be open-hearted, open-minded, and content. It also says:

When the mind confines itself internally, diseases will correspondingly be quieted. When the will has leisure and desires are few, the heart is quiet and not afraid.³ With small desires, thoughts are concentrated. With concentrated thoughts, the mind confines itself internally. When the spirit is confined without abnormalities then the heart is quiet. When the heart is quiet, one's body has a governor. When the body is governed then all parts are active and automatically tend to be normal.

Yǎng Shēn Yāo Jué by Hú Wén Huàn of the Ming Dynasty states:

Abstain from sudden anger to nourish the character. Reduce thinking and worrying to nourish the mind. Use brevity of speech to nourish the qi. Sever thoughts of selfishness to nourish the heart.

This means that avoiding anger, reducing thinking, eliminating worry, speaking conservatively, and severing selfish thoughts are all practical measures for nourishing the heart.

---

³Translator's note—The Chinese character for heart, *xīn*, denotes not only the visceral/physical heart, but also the abstract notion of the mind as seat of consciousness.

The ancients held that "the mind most desires tranquility." They emphasized that "if pleasures and desires are unable to tax one's eyes, environmental excesses and evils cannot beguile the heart." Thought cultivation of this kind encourages people to avoid allowing their imagination to run away with them and to focus their minds on appropriate thoughts. It upholds the maxim that "just thoughts nourish the mind."

In this manner the heart is in an unperturbed state, the mind has no suffering, and the seven affects cannot be harassed; the qi and blood are regulated, harmonious, free and outthrusting, while activities of the viscera and bowels are adjusted, and the dynamic of generation is naturally stable. If one has bursts of joy and bursts of anger, or starts happily and ends bitterly, these all damage essence and qi; when the essence and qi become exhausted and expire then the body breaks down. Especially when doing preventive work for mental abnormalities, physicians in the ancient dynasties emphasized cultivating the heart.

Shòu Shì Xīn Biān by Yóu Shēng Zhōu of the Qing Dynasty includes the following poem on cultivating the heart:

One should know when one's own heart is sick.
When [troubling] thoughts arise, they should be treated.
The heart is only ill when illness arises in the heart.
When the heart is calm, how can illness come?

He thought that only with the heart calm and the qi harmonious, and with distracting thoughts dispelled, might it be possible to have a quiet and stable mind, and thus cultivate health and prevent illness.

If one wishes to create a healthy mental life, first one should nurture and form a love for the people, a love for work, and a love for science, as well as other worthy qualities.[4]

The cerebral cortex in humans is highly malleable. Social skills and subjective motivations are especially important factors that decide the health of the human cerebral cortex. Life cannot

---

[4]Translator's note—"A love" (*rè ài*) and "the people" (*rén mín*) were commonly used political phrases at the time the original authors were writing, and thus must be understood to hold certain connotations.

be eternally tranquil and calm, and not one person is completely happy with the world. Thus, within daily life and work we should build our capacity to endure difficulties and hard work, strengthen the will and not fear difficulties, firmly build a spirit of optimism, and transform negative emotions into positive ones.

These are the best methods and circumstances for altering the activities of the cerebral cortex in the human mind. Facts prove that if a person has a clear challenge and goal, firm conviction, and a strong love for the collective good, then most often he is emotionally stable and optimistic. In contrast, when a person is lazy and idle, or is compelled to do dull, uninteresting work, his emotions can sink and thereby harm his health. Therefore, an appropriate aim for safeguarding and nourishing the mind is to avoid stinting one's capacity. Avoid striving for comfort and avoid idly loafing. This is to prevent oneself from becoming weak and powerless.

In order to maintain a healthy and bountiful mental life, one must have the environment of a good society. Since remote antiquity, human beings have been living and working together, gradually developing reciprocal relations within society, or "social bonds." These ties were quite effective in the development of production, and had an enormous influence on the advances of humanity in later times. Within social bonds individuals always hold closer relationships to certain people. As they mutually assist each other they form nuclear groups. When facing difficulties, emergencies, or times of disaster, these nuclear groups can perform an important support function.

Within mutual social relations, individuals relate to nuclear groups in differing ways; hence the amount of support received during emotionally distressing periods varies from individual to individual. However, the great majority of people still need to maintain a minimum level of social interaction with other people. If it goes below this level, then the prevalence of mental disorders will noticeably increase. Events such as losing a mother in childhood, or disharmony between husband and wife, could cripple one's nuclear group relations, and could be a major factor in emotional damage.

Hans Selye, in *Forty Years of Research on Stress* (1976), had one article that pointed out:

Just as people love themselves, they should love their neighbors and friends the same. This alone is conducive to maintaining interpersonal harmony, withstanding various stimuli, and attaining satisfaction within human relationships.

In a section of *Support Systems and Mental Health in Society* (1981), Caplan pointed out:

Mental disorders could be reduced if patients had effective support from society.

In December of 1974, the city of Darwin, Australia suffered a tornado that destroyed 90% of all residences. Of the 45,000-member population, 50 people lost their lives, and over 30,000 were scattered and separated. When Parker did on-the-spot interviews of these scattered families, he discovered that even under such distressing circumstances, those who were supported by their social group were not psychologically traumatized, whereas those suffering losses in the evacuation who felt they were receiving little social support, soon showed signs of mental disorder. This shows that social support can assuage the degree of mental distress, emotional imbalance, or psychological trauma.

Regarding infants, youth, and the elderly, one should pay attention to mental health concerns for each special group. While nervous personality types have special innate characteristics, they are definitely not fixed and unchangeable. Under the influences of the external environment and individual growth, as well as the influence of regular teaching and training, one can modify the characteristics of nervous personality types. Thus, character development that engenders a high degree of flexibility should start from childhood and develop firmly and steadily. This is the main task of education and a guarantee for preventing illness.

In order to guarantee health of a newborn's body and mind, one should start by tuning and protecting the pregnant mother's mental and psychological state. Especially in the early stages of pregnancy, when the fetus is developing the individual organs and the nervous system, one should strengthen the mother's character, build noble sentiments, and maintain a pleasant mental state. This can influence normal development of the fetus. "Training the fetus" in this way is the beginning of a child's early education. Pavlov said, "To start providing education three days after a baby is born is to have already delayed for three days." This strongly suggests the value of training the fetus.

During infancy and childhood, children primarily have contact with father, mother, and childcare workers. Parents should not spoil their children in a hundred and one ways, nor should they punish indiscriminately. Fathers and mothers are the earliest teachers of children. To be a teacher of children, one should have a proper attitude, and "yes" and "no" should be made clear. Verbal instructions to children make only a slight influence while a realistic example can be a great influence on the development of a child's behavior.

The stage of adolescence is also an important period of development. At this age, contact with the environment becomes more complex, biological change intensifies, and sexual awareness begins to develop. During this time, one should work with a positive approach to open interests and concerns, and encourage the honest attainment of satisfaction. One should stimulate initiative and positiveness, encourage participation in group activities, and support a spirit of collectivism. Moreover, while joining in challenges and overcoming difficulties, youths exercise will power and ambition. As for sex education, it should start during childhood, but during adolescence it is clearly of greater significance. For example, one should give biological and hygienic information on menstruation and spermatorrhea, and proper regard for the opposite sexes should replace mistaken fantasies and ideas.

In old age it is typical for physical capacity to decline. For geriatric patients, there is a mounting risk of development of a variety of disorders, and the risk of all types of mental damage or disorders also increases. Moreover, many health problems of elderly people are intricately interwoven with loneliness in old age, and the psychological effects of a reduced role in society. However, mental deterioration is not absolutely an unavoidable side effect of aging. Arranging for elders to engage in suitable social services and projects can revive their social value and respect, and can reassure them that within the national plan they can still make a contribution. This makes life in later years full of vitality and radiance.

Additionally, a fine mental condition must have the foundation of a strong, healthy body. Therefore, active restraint and prevention of physical diseases, such as infections, trauma, poisoning, and endocrine disturbances, can have positive effects in schizophrenia prevention.

II. MAINTAINING THE CENTRAL NERVOUS SYSTEM

The brain is the physical basis of the psyche, intelligence, and consciousness. A person's will and thoughts, no matter how supersensory they may appear, are always the product of substantive organs. Moreover, the mind itself is then the highest product of that substance. The substantive essence of mental activity is the neural activity of the brain, while the brain is an organ that actualizes and modifies the relationship between the body and its surrounding environment. The brain modifies how the body endures every influence from the outside world, and makes the body capable of maintaining equilibrium in a given environment or in the external world.

Therefore, regarding prevention of schizophrenia and the question of maintaining health, the important point is to protect and strengthen the nervous system, and to reach an equilibrium of cerebral cortex excitement and inhibition. Capacity of the brain is efficiently applied by such means as a lifestyle with rhythms and regulation, adequate and comfortable repose, avoidance of excessive mental distress, prevention of fatigue, and employing active rest.

1. MAINTAINING A BALANCED LIFESTYLE

Regularity and rhythm in life and work has great significance to health. All natural phenomena and life activities have a certain meter or rhythm. Daily work, rest, nourishment, sleep, and exercise should be rationally planned until they form a steady routine. Pavlov used the alternating excitement centers of the cerebral cortex and the theory of dynamic stereotypy to erect basic principles for regulating one's lifestyle routine. The excitatory regions of the cerebral cortex alternate in a way that lets brain cells recuperate, and thereby prevent overexcitement and fatigue. If activities of everyday life are in regulated arrangement, vis-à-vis conditioned reflexes it is possible to develop dynamic stereotypy, and reduce the burden on the nervous system as well as enhance adaptability, while activities of the visceral organs also undergo changes in response. A well-regulated lifestyle should be based on an individual's age, career, home situation, living environment, and other factors of physical health.

The *Inner Canon* points out that we should "eat and drink in moderation, and lead a normal life." Our ancient scholars of health cultivation and disease prevention took guidance from the classical medical saying, "the formal body and the spirit conjoin into one." "Formal body" is all of the body's tissues and organs. "Spirit" is the mind's conscious activities. "The formal body and the spirit conjoin into one" simply means the physical form of the body combines with the spirit-mind allowing the physical form of the body and its capacities to make a unified whole.

In the *Shén Miè Lún* by Fàn Zhěn of the Southern Chao Dynasty, it said:

> The spirit is but physical form; physical form is but the spirit. This is because if the physical form exists, then the spirit exists; if the physical form declines then the mind is extinguished.

Nourishing the mind safeguards the body/form; safeguarding the body then conserves the spirit. The body/form is the residence of the spirit; only when the body is fully suitable can normal mental phenomenon be produced. Methods for cultivation of the body, besides paying attention to eating and drinking in moderation, also must include "leading a normal life." One must adopt a patterned lifestyle with rhythms. *Sù Wèn*, *"Shàng Gǔ Tiān Zhēn Lùn"* says:

> If the body is taxed but not fatigued, the qi is correspondingly

favorable.

This means that if labor and rest are in regularity, the spirit and qi are naturally quiet and favorable. "Leading a normal life" is the path to cultivating health and preventing disease. Excessive taxation and fatigue are harmful to the body; excessive comfort will also generate disease.

2. SLEEP AND TREATMENTS FOR INSOMNIA

Sleep is an important biological phenomenon, as it takes up approximately one third of human life. Sleep allows the body to rest fully; it prevents an organism from becoming exhausted, promotes recovery of strength, increases labor capacity, and is a prerequisite for clear thought. Modern science mostly regards the basic nature of sleep as an inhibition process of higher nervous activity. It is the manifestation of the central nervous system creating a general inhibition.

When the inhibiting process created by the cerebral cortex spreads through the greater part of the cerebral cortex or throughout it, and even goes to the subcortical structure, one then correspondingly enters the state of sleep. During this kind of inhibition process, the nerve cells actively rest, recuperate, and restore depleted functional capacities. At this time they accumulate large quantities of oxygen and other nutritive substances. This prevents exhaustion of nerve cells and possesses a protective nature. Therefore, sleep is a protective inhibition that is of significant importance for the human body.

The quality of sleep is determined not only by duration; the depth of sleep is even more important. Deep, sound sleep is the best, while unsettled, shallow, dream-filled sleep is relatively poor. [If one wants] to make sleep attain the proper duration and depth, one must cultivate a moderate lifestyle and regular sleeping habits. A set time to sleep, and a set time to awaken are fundamental practices of regulated sleep. Factors that assist sleep entry include a calm environment, dimness, and simple sounds. Factors such as light rays, excessive cold or heat, and dampness can cause excitement of the cerebral cortex and prevent dispersion of cortex inhibition. Physical activity has a great influence on sleep. Therefore, all people whose work is predominantly intellectual should seek daily physical exertion.

Insomnia is often an early symptom of schizophrenia and other mental disorders. Preventing insomnia is significant for maintaining health and protecting the strength of the intellect. Insomnia occurs when the normal regulation of higher nervous activity is shattered, causing cerebral excitement and inhibition processes to lose balanced adjustment.

Therefore, when treating insomnia it is important to make the excitement and inhibition processes of the cortex recover a new balance, or to change the abnormal occurrence of poor excitement strength during the daytime, and weak inhibition strength at night. During the daytime one can undertake appropriate physical work or exercise; this makes daytime cerebral cortex activity maintain sufficient excitement such that by evening it naturally turns to inhibition. As the time to sleep approaches, it is appropriate to avoid thinking about problems, to talk little, and to avoid tobacco, alcohol, strong tea, and other stimulants. These can cause the cortex to become excited and prevent sleep. When there are accompanying diseases they should be treated simultaneously.

According to Chinese medicine, insomnia is due to prevalence of one or more of the seven affects. Thus, *Sù Wèn, "Liù Jié Zàng Xiàng Lùn"* says: "The heart is the root of life and the variations in the spirit." The *Sù Wèn, "Kǒu Wèn"* records: "With sorrow and anxiety the heart is stirred."

Zhāng Jǐng Yuè in the Ming Dynasty pointed out:

> *Sleep is rooted in the yin, and the spirit is its governor. When the spirit is quiet then there is sleep; when the spirit is not quiet then there is no sleep.*

Reflecting on this, physicians throughout our ancient dynasties reiterated that "the essence-spirit most desires tranquility." They emphasized "tempering of desires" to make a healthy body and nourish the heart, as well as to prevent diseases from the seven affects.

Regarding "tempering of desires," the essential intent is not to rely on feelings to mold one's temperament, but to have an adaptable nature and contented feelings. Everything should develop from practical circumstances. Properly cultivating health does not at all exclude normal thoughts and desires. However, carnal desire should be tempered in moderation.

Xún Zǐ's *Zhèng Míng Piān* says:

> *Desires are from the affects … desires that [one] cannot let go of, one can seek to temper.*

This means that emotional desires can be tempered with moderation. Although emotional desires have prenatal influences (inherited elements), they can always be constrained by subjective circumstances, and postnatal influences can cause suitable changes.

In addition, since the ancient dynasties there have been many methods of internal cultivation and external cultivation (*nèi gōng* and *wài gōng*)[5] exercise methods that all have the aim of nourishing the heart and quieting the spirit, and are beneficial for preventing and treating diseases of the seven affects. Internal cultivation employs "regulating the heart" in order to nourish the spirit, regulating respiration in order to nourish qi, and regulating the body in order to nourish form.

This actively puts one's whole being into the state of "essence-spirit residing within," which encompasses activities like breathing and consciousness. In this way, within tranquility there is activity. In external cultivation one consciously carries out an ordered routine of movements that are encompassed by focussing the conscious will; thus, within activity there is tranquility. Examples of this are *wŭ qín xì* [the Five Animal exercises], *bā duàn lĭn, tài jí quán,* and so forth.

---

[5]Translator's note—*nèi gōng* and *wài gōng* are two aspects of *qì gōng*—a term for one of the Chinese martial arts more familiar in the West. *Qì gōng* could be literally translated as "working the *qì*" but is more commonly translated as *qì* cultivation. *Nèi gōng* implies working with the internal *qì*, while *wài gōng* implies working with the external qi; *nèi/wài* may be further understood through their yin/yang relationship—internal/external, invisible/visible, quiescent/active.

3. FATIGUE AND ITS PREVENTION

When the human body engages in physical or mental labor and decreased capability for work results, this is called fatigue. It is a biological response of the whole organism. There are many forms of fatigue. One kind has the primary manifestation of systematic physical fatigue; often there are special subjective feelings such as weariness or reluctance to engage in physical activity. Another kind of fatigue is primarily mental fatigue, which frequently is marked by dizziness, headache, and feeling of distention in the head,[6] weakness throughout the body, craving for sleep or else insomnia, a tendency to irritability, and flaccidity of muscles. In the production of fatigue, no matter whether it is fatigue of the physical body or of mental power, the central nervous system plays a predominant role.

Fatigue is a transient biological phenomenon. It is a kind of warning to the organism. No matter whether it is the physical or mental energy that is fatigued, the cerebral cortex is functioning protectively. It shows that brain cells need rest. During daytime brain cells are ceaselessly damaged by activity, yet concurrently there is recovery. Sleep during the nighttime allows damage reparations to be completed. If fatigue as a biological phenomenon persists without complete recovery for a prolonged time, then balance is destroyed between damage and repair. An accumulation of fatigue, or what is simply named "excessive taxation," can result.

Schizophrenia occurs when the central nervous system malfunctions. Cells of the cerebral cortex, through conditioned reflexes, carry out analysis and summarization on the one hand, while on the other hand they analyze and synthesize stimuli from every sector of the organism, and maintain a balanced relationship between the organism and the environment. This assures that the internal and external environments of the organism are unified. Not only is this activity extremely intricate, but the cerebral cortex cells that are involved are unusually sensitive

---

[6]Translator's note—A feeling of pressure and discomfort in the head. Distention in the head is usually caused by external contraction of dampness evil, or non-elimination of summerheat-warmth evil. It is variously treated by resolving the exterior, clearing heat, repelling foulness, and transforming dampness.

and fragile. Thus, a sudden strong excitement, or a prolonged period of excitement conflicting with inhibition, can damage the cells of the cerebral cortex.

A principle of treatment for schizophrenia is to protect the cells of the cerebral cortex, and assist recovery of normal capacity. Looking at it in this way, paying attention to sleep and rest is important for prevention of schizophrenia.

4. EMPLOYING ACTIVE REST

By positing that the central nervous system has a guiding role in the mechanism of fatigue or the mechanism by which fatigue arises, we can then explain the role of functional states of the central nervous system in the development of and recovery from fatigue.

Literature from abroad has pointed out, "Weariness or lack of interest in work is an emotional factor that can create fatigue," which underscores the easily understood concept of central nervous system fatigue. In preventing fatigue, the first thing is for the patient to develop his or her subjective capabilities, gain faith in working for humanity, love his or her work, and overcome negative psychological factors. Secondarily one should pay attention to scheduling work and rest. As there is a limit to how much work a person can do, one should adopt biological laws to unify work and rest in a rhythm. Rest is for the sake of maximum recovery of work capacity. Working hours should not be too long, and should be interspersed with breaks. These customs are effective for [promoting] recovery of the biological functions of the cortex cells and physical strength.

The Russian physiologist Shcherov[7] experimented on styles of rest. He discovered that when a human body has a group of muscles which has already worked to fatigue, if one rests only that group of muscles for a short period while working another

---

[7]Translator's note—It is hard to say exactly who was this Russian physiologist. The characters used to indicate his surname are pronounced "Xie Qie Ruo Fu." According to Russian speakers, the Russian surname that likely corresponds is Shcherov. However, we could not locate any sources that positively identified a Russian physiologist who would have done this research.

group of muscles, then fatigue is diminished most rapidly. This illuminates how the style of active rest is superior to passive rest.

From the viewpoint of biology, when we are engaged in mental or physical labor, the internal regions of the body and the surrounding environment produce a vast number of stimulations. These excite cells in the corresponding regions of the cerebral cortex, while cells in other unrelated regions are at rest. When one changes to another kind of labor, making the worked organs rest and the unworked organs active, excitement of cerebral cortex cells enter a rotation. Passive rest indicates sitting, lying, or another passive rest or sleep. The two kinds of rest, active and passive, can be coordinated and interchanged. Styles of rest should be individually suited to circumstances such as career, age, health status, and lifestyle.

Going from one mental activity to another kind of mental activity is also a method for resting. Chatting and jovial conversation is a kind of rest; it is a manifestation of happiness and high spirits that can allow someone to break away from serious thoughts and to feel relaxed emotionally, and it can enhance the function of the nervous system. Rest combined with cultural recreation and physical exercise is another positive method that stimulates the mind. For those who engage in mental work that involves distress on the nervous system, daily engagement in a fixed period of physical exertion or athletic activity not only creates the effect of an active rest, it also deepens sleep. Thus, it both directly and indirectly helps recovery from fatigue.

In addition, one should also create pleasant, restful surroundings by making good use of fresh air and sunshine. Vocational environments can be improved by reducing undesirable stimulations, such as eliminating annoying noises and vibrations.

The ancient Chinese school of cultivating health and preventing disease was developed and built upon the foundation and theories from traditional medicine and its applications. It is inseparable from what traditional medical sciences consider to be the basic, necessary elements, or what the ancient scholars of cultivating health called the "three internal jewels"—essence, qi, and spirit.

These are the ingredients of a vital organism, as well as the human body's force for activity. Within the triad of essence, qi, and spirit, qi serves as the foundation of essence and spirit. Only upon the basis of qi's substantive activity can there then be the production/generation of essence, and functions of the spirit. The triad of essence, qi, and spirit are cyclically, mutually converting. This conversion process is the result of the movement and evolution of qi in all its different forms. Qi is the root and stem of essence and spirit; if qi is sufficient then essence is sufficient; if qi is vacuous then essence is vacuous. Only when essence and qi are effulgent and exuberant can essence and spirit be vigorous.

An essential aspect of cultivating health is that one must accumulate qi to generate essence, and accumulate essence to form the spirit. Thus, the *Pí Wèi Lùn* by Lǐ Dōng Yuán of the Jin Dynasty states:

> Qi is the ancestor of the spirit; essence is the son of qi. Qi is the root and stem of essence and spirit.

The traditional Chinese school of cultivating health, while using numerous methods that have centuries of history, consistently emphasizes safeguarding essence, qi, and spirit. The ancients summed this up in the phrase, "safeguard essence, cultivate bountiful qi, and nourish the spirit." They felt that to cultivate health, "qi and blood most desire movement, and essence and mind most desire tranquility."

This idea naturally combines tranquility and movement, and practically encompasses what modern science promotes as the active resting form. When the ancients proclaimed that "qi and blood most desire movement," they simultaneously emphasized balance between work and rest. This is because excessive taxation consumes qi, advances to damage essence, and quells the spirit.

Thus, *Sù Wèn*, "*Shàng Gǔ Tiān Zhēn Lùn*" states: "The body should be taxed but not exhausted." *Bèi Jí Qiān Jīn Yào Fāng* by Sūn Sī Miǎo in the Tang Dynasty states: "In the path of cultivating health, frequently desire slight taxation." *Bào Pǔ Zǐ* by Gé

Hóng in the Jin Dynasty states: "The body desires constant taxation ... taxation not exceeding an extreme."

From these quotations we can know that scholars in our ancient dynasties understood the nature of work and rest and their scientific arrangement. Though their insights are quite old, they are fundamentally similar to those held today.

III. Emphasis on Early Diagnosis and Treatment

An important link in the work to prevent schizophrenia is identifying the disorder, making a diagnosis, and giving suitable treatment as early as possible. This can prevent the disorder from developing to a more serious, chronic stage. The earlier the disease is diagnosed, the more effective and speedier the treatment will be, and the sooner the patient will be restored to health. In contrast, chronic cases are more difficult, and require longer treatment, often with less effective results.

Consequently, research on the early stage symptoms of schizophrenia has a special, practical importance. For example, when the early stage of schizophrenia appears as compulsive neurosis, a wonderful result is likely if it is verified early and treated suitably. In addition, there are early signs of mental disorders that can be discovered during infancy and childhood. For example, susceptibility to irritation and fatigue, irrational fears, unquiet sleep, and various forms of convulsions frequently portend that a serious illness is just beginning and will require attention and correction as soon as possible.

Modern treatment therapies for schizophrenia are appropriate for early stages and can achieve high cure rates. The professional literature shows that treatment is twice as effective in the first year as in the second year. If treatment is required beyond a few months, there are serious concerns for the prognosis. Early diagnosis and treatment have the same importance for all mental disorders. By training proficient medical workers and constantly upgrading knowledge of mental health among the people, early diagnosis, treatment, and recovery are achievable goals.

When a schizophrenia patient passes from an acute state into clinical recuperation, they have low resistance. In extreme cases, relatively mild stimuli can be sufficient to cause mental activity to relapse into a schizoid state. Moreover, during clinical recuperation the possibility of lapsing into a chronic condition still exists. For these reasons, during the recuperative stage the body's defensive forces should be fortified. Primarily we should provide the patient with adequate and effective therapy to consolidate the cure.

After the patient has received treatment, they should also have appropriate vocational and exercise therapy, ample sleep and rest, and avoidance of emotional stress or other harmful influences from their daily environment. These measures serve to increase the strength of the nervous system and prevent relapse or entry into a long-term, chronic state.

~ CHAPTER FIVE ~
TREATMENTS

SCHIZOPHRENIA IS A CHRONIC, progressive disorder. In the initial stage, most cases are latent, while only a small number take an acute or subacute form. No matter whether the disorder arises slowly or rapidly, it usually presents with a progressively developing nature. The duration of illness may span a few months, a few years, or even longer. (The duration of disease must be a minimum of three months, including at least one month's duration of psychosis.)[1]

If appropriate treatment is not given, then in the end the great majority of patients tend toward mental decline, and dementia occurs. When organic changes develop in the brain, then the possibility of recovery is extremely slight.

I. TREATMENTS BASED ON THE AUTHORS' EXPERIENCE

Acupuncture and moxibustion produce good effects in the treatment of schizophrenia. In the context of Chinese medical thought,

---

[1]Translator's note—The history of schizophrenia is filled with debates about the definition of schizophrenia. Because it is so hard to define, what is accepted as the definition changes from country to country and from time to time. *Merch's Manual* has this to say about the diagnosis of schizophrenia: "According to *Diagnostic and Statistical Manual of Mental Disorders, Fourth Edition (DSM-IV)*, two or more characteristic symptoms (delusions, hallucinations, disorganized speech, disorganized behavior, negative symptoms) for a significant portion of a one-month period are required for the diagnosis, and prodromal or attenuated signs of illness with social, occupational, or self-care impairments must be evident for a six-month period that includes one month of active symptoms."

this disorder falls within the scope of mania-withdrawal *(diān kuáng)*. The use of acupuncture and moxibustion for treatment of schizophrenia has greatly advanced in recent years.

In establishing acupuncture treatment principles, treating qi is the root consideration. The basic action of acupuncture is to harmonize the qi and blood, and course and free the channels and network vessels. From the viewpoint of modern science, acupuncture produces its regulating effect through the central nervous system especially by influencing cerebral cortex function, by adjusting activities of the vegetative nervous system, and by altering the activity level of endocrine glands.

Thus, what Chinese physicians regard as mania-withdrawal, or disharmony of qi and blood with phlegm and fire harassing the heart, is what Western physicians refer to as schizophrenia resulting from functional disorder of the cerebral cortex. Acupuncture is an excellent treatment for this disorder.

We have differentiated two types: mania *(kuáng)* disease type and withdrawal *(diān)* disease type. These types are founded upon the special symptoms that patients have presented in our clinical experience of treating this disorder.

1. TREATMENTS FOR MANIA *(KUÁNG)* DISEASE TYPE—EXCITATORY STATE

PATTERN IDENTIFICATION

Mania is ascribed to yang, and is generally repletion. The onset of disease is rather rapid. At first a rash and impatient nature is evidenced; the mind is vexed and irascible. The patient has insomnia and reduced food intake. Then there follows red face and ears, and an angry look from both eyes. Patients feel disquieted when sitting or lying; they make a ceaseless din, curse and hit people, speak in illogical sequence, and have constipation. They may also wreak destruction and harm themselves, run recklessly everywhere, throw off their clothes and go around naked, exhibit extraordinary physical strength, and not alter their [strange] behavior for either family or strangers.[2] In mania patients the tongue body is red or purple, the tongue fur is yellow and thick, or yellow and slippery, while the pulse reading is surging and large, or stringlike and slippery.

The *Inner Canon* states, "Excessive agitation and mania are all ascribed to fire." This pathomechanism is operant in most mania patterns. Depressed fire forms phlegm, and harasses the heart and mind above. When the spirit light is without a ruler, then disease occurs. Thus, appropriate treatment is primarily governed by clearing heat, flushing phlegm, and settling the heart.

PRIMARY POINT SELECTION

[Use] bilateral PC-7 (*dà líng*), bilateral HT-7 (*shén mén*), bilateral LI-11 (*qū chí*), bilateral ST-40 (*fēng lóng*), and GV-16 (*fēng fǔ*). In each treatment, employ all these points while combining appropriate symptomatic points.

On the basis of a patient's individual symptoms, one may make additions such as:

Auditory hallucinations	GB-2 (*tīng huì*) and TB-17 (*yì fēng*).
Visual hallucinations	BL-1 (*jīng míng*) and M-HN-8 (*qiú hòu*)
Unclear spirit-mind	GV-26 (*rén zhōng*) and KI-1 (*yǒng quǎn*)
Taciturnity	GV-15 (*yǎ mén*) and CV-23 (*lián quán*)
Excessive speech	GB-20 (*fēng chí*).

MANIPULATION TECHNIQUE

[The patient should] assume a recumbent posture for needling. When performing the acupuncture manipulation, the needle must have a rotational draining method with rapid rotation and a wide arc. The best results are achieved when rotation is continued until the patient has a dazed-like desire to sleep.

---

[2]Translator's note—See page 9 for an explanation regarding this phrase.

MEANING OF THE FORMULA

In this type of patient, anger causes the liver and gallbladder qi to counterflow, leading qi, fire, phlegm, and turbidity to upwardly harass the spirit light. Thus, points such as HT-7 (shén mén), PC-7 (dà líng), and LI-11 (qū chí) are selected to drain heat evils from the shào yīn heart, jué yīn pericardium, and yáng míng large intestine channels. ST-40 (fēng lóng) assists in transforming phlegm and GV-16 (fēng fǔ) arouses the brain. This establishes a governor for the spirit light, which automatically resolves mania and delirium.

CHINESE MEDICINALS

This foundational acupuncture treatment can be enhanced at the practitioner's discretion with a prescription of Chinese medicinals, as it is often helpful for this type of patient. In addition to needling one could give a medicinal agent decoction with 30 grams each of dried/fresh rehmannia (shēng dì) and bamboo shavings (zhú rú), administered with two Purple Snow Elixir Pills (Zǐ Xuě Dān), twice daily. This clears heat and flushes phlegm, cools blood, and dissipates stasis.

CASE HISTORY

Patient: Chen XX, male, age 26, party member.

From his father's account, the patient's disposition had been of a quiet nature since childhood. He treated people honestly, got along well with his brothers and sisters, and was obedient to his parents. While attending school he was often at the top of his class.

After the liberation of Hang Zhou he studied energetically and worked sincerely. Later one of his co-workers publicly suspected him of corrupt acts prior to the Liberation, and this led him to develop emotional tension and insomnia. He was fidgety the whole day, talked ceaselessly and had flailing limbs. He would force others to hear him through, and if they did not go along, he would start to strike them. He was taken to a mental hospital and diagnosed as having schizophrenia. He received chlorpromazine and other drug treatments. However, even after more than ten days had passed he was still unable to sleep calmly. The condition was unabated and worsening. At that time his father brought him specifically for acupuncture treatment.

<u>INITIAL EXAMINATION, JUNE 10</u>

The patient had a stalwart build, red face and ears, and an angry stare in both eyes; he had no thought of food, and was constipated. Although he had been without sleep for ten days, his essence-spirit was not weary. The tongue was red with a yellow fur; the pulse reading was stringlike and slippery. The disease was from unrelenting depression and anger that was not drained causing liver depression to transform into fire and phlegm-heat to harass the heart, giving rise to mania pattern.

The treatment plan was to resolve depression and drain fire, transform phlegm, and settle the heart. After his father took measures to convince him, the patient consented to acupuncture therapy.

POINT SELECTION:

GV-16 (*fēng fǔ*) and GB-20 (*fēng chí*) were first needled, followed by LI-11 (*qū chí*) and ST-40 (*fēng lóng*); all points had rotating, draining manipulation. Each point had hand-needle stimulation for one to two minutes, and no needles were retained. Next HT-7 (*shén mén*) and PC-7 (*dà líng*) were also needled with rotating, draining manipulation; needles were retained at both locations and rotation was performed in alternation. About five minutes later the patient had the urge to sleep, so the needles were left in to maintain needle sensation. Approximately two minutes later the patient fell asleep on the examination table, and slept for almost one hour.

<u>SECOND EXAMINATION, JUNE 11</u>

The patient was again accompanied by his father, who reported that after returning home from the acupuncture treatment on the previous day the symptoms of irritability and excitability had greatly abated. The patient spoke less, moved his bowels during the night, and was even able to get to sleep; he was calmer emotionally. At the clinic on this day, symptoms such as his red eyes and angry expression were noticeably lessened.

POINT SELECTION:

The manipulation technique was the same as the preceding day, yet in this treatment the patient was more sensitive to the needling, and felt that the needles were hard to endure. Moreover, he had no inclination to sleep.

THIRD EXAMINATION, 12 JUNE

The father reported that after returning home from acupuncture treatment the previous day, all was well. The patient's appetite had returned to normal, but he did not wish to speak much. At night he had slept very soundly, and today he was interacting with people, handling objects, and speaking and behaving just as he did before the illness. His spirits were excellent. The stringlike pulse had relaxed, and the tongue fur was scant and clear. He was encouraged to consolidate the therapeutic result with more acupuncture. The previous formula was used again.

POINT SELECTION:

Bilateral HT-7 (shén mén), bilateral PC-7 (dà líng), bilateral LI-11 (qū chí), bilateral ST-40 (fēng lóng), and GV-16 (fēng fǔ).

MANIPULATION TECHNIQUE:

The points above were all needled with rotation draining method, and with no retention. From this time forth acupuncture was discontinued for observation. Follow-up examinations over several years showed that everything was normal and the patient had no relapses.

2. TREATMENT FOR WITHDRAWAL (DIĀN) DISEASE TYPE—MELANCHOLIA CONDITION

PATTERN IDENTIFICATION

The withdrawal disease type is ascribed to yin and is generally a vacuity with repletion complication. Normally the onset of disease is slow, and often one first sees emotional sadness, depressed spirits, insomnia, doubtfulness, and [excessive] thinking. If it continues, there is a cold, indifferent expression, or patients will mutter to themselves. Their speech lacks logical sequence, or their spirit and frame of mind are as if entranced. At times sad while at other times happy, they weep and laugh abnormally. They have no sense of hygiene, and no thought of food. Withdrawal patients have nonsensical thoughts that can be filled with doubt and hesitations, and they are easily frightened. The tongue body is pale red; the tongue fur is white and thick, or white and slimy. The pulse is stringlike and fine, or slippery.

TREATMENT PRINCIPLES

The pathomechanism of withdrawal is usually depressed stagnant liver qi, spleen qi with loss of movement, and congealing fluids that transform into turbid phlegm. Thus, clouding of the spirit-light results in illness. Therefore, treatment should resolve depression of liver qi, transform phlegm, and quiet the spirit.

POINT SELECTION

The primary points employed are bilateral GB-20 (fēng chí), bilateral BL-18 (gān shū), bilateral BL-20 (pí shū), bilateral ST-40 (fēng lóng), bilateral BL-15 (xīn shū), and bilateral HT-7 (shén mén). All points are used in every treatment. For additional symptomatic points, refer to the mania disease type (p. 57).

MANIPULATION TECHNIQUE

Have the patient assume a recumbent posture for needling. Regarding the acupuncture manipulation, all points should have even supplementation, even draining method, except for using lifting and thrusting draining method on the back points.

MEANING OF THE FORMULA

Patients of this type are mostly seen to have excessive thinking and unattained goals. The result is liver depression and spleen vacuity, gathering humor that forms phlegm, upward counter-flow of phlegm and qi, and abnormal spirit-light; this forms withdrawal disease. Thus, GB-20 (*fēng chí*), BL-18 (*gān shū*), BL-20 (*pí shū*), and ST-40 (*fēng lóng*) are selected to course liver depression, move spleen qi, and transform phlegm and turbidity to treat the root. HT-7 (*shén mén*) and BL-15 (*xīn shū*) are selected to open the heart orifices and revive the spirit-light. By thus resolving depression, withdrawal is automatically cured.

CHINESE MEDICINALS

On the basis of the patient's tongue fur and appetite, one can distinguish two types: "the simple type," and the "complex type." In patients of the simple type, the tongue fur is thin and clear, or thin and white, while the appetite for food is often normal. It is suitable to use a modified Heart Settling Elixir (*Zhèn Xīn Dān*) prescription for treatment:

cooked rehmannia (*shú dì*)	cinnabar-coated root poria (*chén fú shén*)
codonopsis (*dǎng shēn*)	
asparagus (*tiān dōng*)	agrimony (*qīng lóng yá*)
ophiopogon (*mài dōng*)	schisandra (*wǔ wèi zǐ*)
dioscorea (*huái shān yào*)	polygala (*yuǎn zhì*)
spiny jujube (*suān zǎo rén*)	lodestone (*líng cí shí*)

The original formula also has cinnamon bark (*ròu guì*), poria (*fú líng*), and plantago seed (*chē qián zǐ*), but not lodestone (*líng cí shí*).

In patients of the "complex type," the tongue fur is thin and slimy, or thick and slimy, and frequently there is torpid stomach intake. It is suitable to employ [a modified] Ten Ingredients Gallbladder Warming Decoction (*Shí Wèi Wēn Dǎn Tāng*) [consisting of the following ingredients]:

| ginger[-processed] pinellia *(jiāng bàn xià)* poria *(fú líng)* codonopsis *(dǎng shēn)* agrimony *(lóng yá)* dried/fresh rehmannia *(shēng dì)* | spiny jujube *(suān zǎo rén)* tangerine peel *(chén pí)* polygala *(yuǎn zhì)* schisandra *(wǔ wèi zǐ)* unripe bitter orange *(zhǐ shí)* |

The original formula also had licorice *(gān cǎo)*, and did not have agrimony *(lóng yá)*. Moreover, the cooked rehmannia in the original formula was changed to dried/fresh rehmannia.

The primary formulas given above can be modified as follows: if the condition is accompanied with emotional sadness that leads to weeping and tears, one can additionally use Licorice, Wheat, and Jujube Decoction *(Gān Mài Dà Zǎo Tāng)*. For serious head clouding and pain, add mother-of-pearl *(zhēn zhū mǔ)*; for loss of appetite, add anomalous artemisia *(liú jì nú)*; for thoracic oppression and ribside pain, abdominal distension with fullness, and frequent belching, add poncirus *(gǒu jú lǐ)* and cyperus *(zhì xiāng fù)*.

CASE HISTORY

Patient: Jiang XX, female, age 25, worker.

The patient grew up as an only child and from infancy was deeply affected by her parents' doting. During the Cultural Revolution her parents were persecuted, so after junior high graduation she was unable to continue her schooling. She was good-natured, timid, and very obedient. She avoided arguments, and if she encountered conflict preferred to suffer on her own. Because she was so honest and had such a gentle personality, during schooling she was easily bullied by classmates and frequently returned home crying.

During summer vacation in her twentieth year, she accompanied her mother on a journey to a distant place to visit relatives. While fatigued from traveling she received a great fright and spent the whole night in terror and intense emotional distress.

Afterwards she was depressed throughout the day, and her essence-spirit was dull. The patient spoke sparingly, had a dull shine in her eyes, a pale, indifferent expression, and sleeplessness through the night. After two months she was admitted to a mental hospital and was diagnosed as having schizophrenia. By taking chlorpromazine, amitriptyline, and other medications for half a year, the condition improved and she was discharged from the hospital.

Four years later someone introduced a boyfriend. After getting to know each other they found themselves to be emotionally compatible, and developed a very close relationship. Later, on learning that she had been in a mental hospital, the boyfriend distanced himself and broke off the relationship.[3]

This led to bitter sadness and depressed emotions. She was unhappy and in low spirits during waking hours, and unable to sleep at night. Subsequently she showed abnormal spirit-mind manifestations, a cold, indifferent expression, reduced physical movements, and a propensity to weep. The patient was admitted to a mental health hospital again, and after three months of treatment there was still no improvement. When she was given electric shock therapy, her mother felt it was too horrible to watch. She demanded discharge from the mental hospital and sought acupuncture therapy at our clinic.

INITIAL EXAMINATION: 1 SEPTEMBER

The patient's mother accompanied her for examination, and explained that at night the patient was unable to sleep; if she slept, she awoke in fear. She was frightened, disquieted, and had a poor appetite.

The patient's expression was cold and indifferent. Her eyes were dull, and she did not answer questions. With repetitive interrogation, both eyes shed tears. She was sorrowful, weepy, and moved slowly. The pulse was stringlike and fine; the tongue coating was thin and slimy. The illness was diagnosed as the result of

---

[3]Translator's note—Chinese custom implies that such a relationship most likely would lead to marriage. Thus the non-Chinese reader should understand that what the patient experienced was not just the loss of another boyfriend, but a major humiliation.

depressed and stagnant liver qi, non-upbearing of spleen qi, and fluids congealing and gathering, transforming to phlegm and turbidity, thus clouding the spirit-light and manifesting as withdrawal disease.

POINT SELECTION:

Bilateral GB-20 (*fēng chí*), bilateral BL-18 (*gān shū*), bilateral BL-20 (*pí shū*), bilateral BL-15 (*xīn shū*), bilateral HT-7 (*shén mén*), and bilateral ST-40 (*fēng lóng*) [were selected]. Daily acupuncture was prescribed, one course of ten treatments. For all points, even-supplementation, even-draining manipulation [technique] was applied. All the needles were spun for one or two minutes and were not retained.

SECOND EXAMINATION: 2 SEPTEMBER

After acupuncture the day before there was no discernible change in the patient's condition. Points selected and manipulations were the same as the day before.

THIRD EXAMINATION: 3 SEPTEMBER

The preceding night the patient had been able to fall asleep, and her fright and fear were greatly reduced. Other symptoms were the same as before. Acupuncture was continued with the original prescription.

FOURTH EXAMINATION: 4 SEPTEMBER

The patient's nighttime sleep had become deeper, and had continued until the sky was bright. Acupuncture was continued with the original prescription.

FIFTH EXAMINATION: 5 SEPTEMBER

Nighttime sleep was still good. Today the patient's eyes had gained vigor. She responded to questions and was even able to talk about her illness. At this time her sorrowful and tearful demeanor was no longer apparent. Acupuncture was continued with the original prescription.

SIXTH EXAMINATION: 6 SEPTEMBER

The patient's emotions had returned to normal. She herself reported that at night her sleep was sound, with no incidence of waking up frightened, and the taste of food and drink was appealing. Acupuncture therapy was continued with the same prescription.

<u>SEVENTH EXAMINATION: 7 SEPTEMBER</u>

The patient's condition continued to show improvement. She was emotionally cheerful, and was in a normal state of mind. She talked and laughed freely, and independently betook herself to the treatment bed to await acupuncture. Acupuncture was continued with the original prescription.

For consolidation of therapeutic results, this patient completed the initial course of 10 sessions of acupuncture therapy, with no adjustments in the points selected or the needling manipulations. The patient was then advised to discontinue acupuncture for two weeks of observation. As her circumstances were normal, she required no further acupuncture. From that time forward, follow-up observations were made for five years. They showed that in the year following acupuncture the patient was married and gave birth to a baby girl. Her happy disposition and cheerful spirit remained constant.

3. SYMPTOMATIC TREATMENTS FOR WITHDRAWAL AND MANIA PATTERNS

The *Nán Jīng, "Twenty-Second Difficulty"* says:

> In patients with weighted yang there is mania; in patients with weighted yin there is withdrawal.

We hold the opinion that in diagnosing mania and withdrawal one must first differentiate yin and yang to clarify what is most important. Following that, the withdrawal and mania varieties of schizophrenia disorders belong to the same conflict within one entity.

Moreover, in accord with given circumstances one may transform into the other. Just as it is stated in *Elementary Questions, "Mài Jiě"*:

> In one who is said to desire staying alone behind closed doors and windows, there is mutual contention of yin and yang. Yang is at

the extreme and yin is exuberant. Thus they like to close the doors and stay put. In those who are said to desire to climb to a high place and sing out, or to throw off their clothes and run amok, the yin and yang repeatedly engage in struggle and externally concentrate in yang, thus making them throw off their clothes and run amok.

The phenomenon of "tranquil yin" and "agitated yang" patterns transforming into one another occurs frequently in schizophrenic disorders. *Yī Xué Zhōng Zhòng Cān Xī Lù* by Zhāng Xī Chún in the Qing Dynasty pointed out:

Generally, when this disease originates, there is first a slight show of withdrawal which then develops into mania. When mania is enduring and uncured, it also gradually forms withdrawal, or in its extreme may form complete loss of perception.

Thus, yin-withdrawal and yang-mania within schizophrenic disorders are mutually opposite, as well as a mutually unified pair of basic types. In view of this relationship, after first treating the diagnosed conformation, one should then emphasize treating symptoms, i.e., the symptoms that mania and withdrawal frequently hold in common.

A. INSOMNIA

Insomnia is common to all kinds of mental disorders, is the most commonly seen symptom, and is moreover a symptom from the earliest stages of schizophrenia. To address the problem of insomnia, one should first give psychological therapy aimed directly at the patient's individual circumstances. That is, verbal instruction should provide guidance that will reduce mental burdens and increase the strength of belief in treatment.

Additionally, one can counsel patients about general methods for preventing insomnia. At bedtime, insomniacs should avoid thinking of problems and stop trying to will themselves to sleep; [they should] also abstain from food or drink that is excessive in quantity or stimulating in nature before trying to sleep.

POINT SELECTION

For acupuncture therapy one can use: Bilateral HT-7 (shén mén), bilateral GB-20 (fēng chí), and bilateral LI-4 (hé gǔ).

MANIPULATION

Have the patient assume a sitting or supine posture during treatment. Employ a rotational draining method. In general do not retain needles; however, for HT-7 (shén mén) and LI-4 (hé gǔ), seek a needle sensation that radiates to above the elbow. The needle sensation on GB-20 (fēng chí) should extend to the forehead and temple region. If the condition of the disease is severe, or if radiation of needle sensation is not satisfying, then retain the needles for thirty minutes. Needle daily or on alternate days with ten to fifteen treatments comprising one course.

MEANING OF THE FORMULA

The heart is the governing ruler of the whole body. All speech, movement, will, and thought are controlled by the heart. The heart also governs blood and stores the spirit. When blood is vacuous and fire harasses, the spirit fails to keep to its abode, giving rise to vexation, agitation, and insomnia. Therefore the source point of the heart channel, HT-7 (shén mén), is selected to quiet the spirit.

The gallbladder governs decision. When heart blood is insufficient and the gallbladder is deprived of nourishment, then the ministerial fire joins in, further exacerbating the causes of insomnia.

The ancients said that if one cannot sleep at night, if one awakens frightened after scant sleep and turns side-to-side restlessly, then the treatment should be addressed to the shào yáng. Thus GB-20 (fēng chí) assists by coursing and rectifying the gallbladder channel. Moreover, GB-20 (fēng chí) is the meeting point of the hand and foot shào yáng with the yang springing vessel. It can simultaneously treat this yang springing vessel symptom: "When eye qi is not nurtured, then the eyes do not close," such as in insomnia. This is a fortunate coincidence. LI-4 (hé gǔ), the source point of the large intestine channel, is also enjoined for clearing and rectifying fire from all orifices of the head and face. It thereby relaxes and relieves headache, dizziness, tinnitus, and so forth, and has many benefits that improve sleep.

COMMENT

[Following this method of acupuncture treatment] we did electroencephalograms with sleep as the target of observation. We used this technique in clinical research on 23 cases of patients who had been ineffectively treated for insomnia with both Western drugs and Chinese medicinals. The result was that 14 cases recovered, eight cases showed improvement, and one case showed no change. The overall effectiveness rate was 95%. After needling for one course of treatment, the EEG changes for the effectively treated patients showed lower alpha numbers, decreased alpha rate, and lowered alpha wave amplitude. There was even a gradual increase of Q waves. This suggests that acupuncture has a marked effect on brain waves. Perhaps needling the three points explained above produced the result of increasing active inhibition by affecting the higher nervous system.

B. SYMPTOMS OF REFUSAL OF FOOD

Schizophrenic patients frequently refuse food. The causes are quite numerous. For example, people who are self-incriminating delusives often believe that since they are guilty of the most heinous crimes they do not deserve food or drink, and therefore they fast. When patients have delusions of persecution, they may suspect that foods have poison in them, and [thus] will not dare to consume them. Patients with hyperexcitation can also refuse food. Patients with heavy conflicts in their thoughts can ponder over and over what to eat first, and through irresolution make no final decision. Stuporous patients do not eat or drink because of the general cessation of physical movement.

The procedures for management of refusal of food depend on the special circumstances of each case. Except for stuporous patients, one should first provide guidance and explanations that help the patient understand the importance of nutrition for the body. For suspicious patients, someone could first eat a small portion of the food to relieve the patient's concerns. For certain patients, once they have repeatedly become starvingly hungry, one can use delicious dishes or fruits to entice them into eating. For patients with delusions of guilt, one may set out food for them, and allow them to eat on their own when no one else is around.

POINT SELECTION

For acupuncture one could use the following: Bilateral PC-6 *(nèi guān)*, bilateral TB-17 *(yì fēng)*, bilateral BL-18 *(gān shū)*, and bilateral BL-20 *(pí shū)*. For patients of stuporous type, select CV-23 *(lián quán)*, CV-22 *(tiān tú)*, and bilateral KI-1 *(yǒng quǎn)*.

MANIPULATION TECHNIQUE

Have the patient assume a recumbent posture for needling. Perform even supplementing, even draining manipulation on the first four points; employ rotational draining method on the latter three points (in stuporous patients). In most cases do not retain the needles. Administer acupuncture treatments once or twice daily.

MEANING OF THE FORMULA

The heart stores the spirit, prolonged thought wears the spirit, and when disease in the mother affects the child, there is damage to the spleen. Also, the liver governs fright; fright damages the liver. In prolonged circumstances the wind stirs and the phlegm ascends, phlegm obstructs the clear orifices, and the results are manifestations of eccentricity, suspiciousness, refusal of food, and other mental conditions. These can directly develop into the stuporous conditions of mutism and dementedly standing (or sitting) without moving.

Therefore, select PC-6 *(nèi guān)* (the river point of the hand *jué yīn* pericardium channel) to open the orifices of the heart; choose TB-17 *(yì fēng)* to settle fright and extinguish wind;

employ BL-18 *(gān shū)* and BL-20 *(pí shū)* for orderly reaching of liver wood, while moving the spleen and transforming phlegm.

If the disease progresses for many days then phlegm and fire gather together, the humor becomes desiccated, and liquids are damaged, so there is stupor or mania. At that point use CV-23 *(lián quán)* or CV-22 *(tiān tú)* to sweep phlegm and open orifices; meanwhile, KI-1 *(yǒng quǎn)* clears fire and rouses the spirit, such that this disease is resolved.

COMMENT

Refusal of food in mental patients is commonly the result of depressed and obstructing phlegm and heat. Usually there are symptoms of upward closure (phlegm stagnation and dull spirit), downward blockage [constipation], and qi binding. Besides using acupuncture therapy, one may with discretion apply Chinese medicinal agents such as Phlegm Abducting Decoction *(Dǎo Tán Tāng)* and Major Qi-Coordinating Decoction *(Dà Chéng Qì Tāng)*, with variations. These formulas clear fire and transform phlegm, as well as free the bowels and discharge evils, to resolve the symptoms at an early stage.

C. HALLUCINATIONS AND DELUSIONS

Hallucinations and delusions are common symptoms in schizophrenic patients. Patients [can] have profuse delusions and hallucinations; because the two symptoms are closely related and mutually influencing, they normally manifest as a singular entity. For example, patients with delusions of reference or delusions of persecution may simultaneously have auditory hallucinations. The hallucinations that a patient hears may make them become even more set on their delusionary thoughts. It is also possible that delusions can reinforce auditory hallucinations, and thereby make a disorder more critical. In addition to using common psychotherapy, one can employ the following acupuncture therapy.

POINT SELECTION

Bilateral GB-20 (*fēng chí*), bilateral GB-2 (*tīng huì*), and bilateral LR-3 (*tài chōng*).

MANIPULATION

Have the patient assume a recumbent posture for needling. Employ rotational draining method with 15 to 30 minutes of needle retention. In severe cases one may use electroacupuncture. Do one acupuncture treatment daily.

MEANING OF THE FORMULA

Hallucinations and delusions are usually from liver and gallbladder fire encroaching upward, resulting in harassment of the heart and spirit. Therefore, select GB-20 (*fēng chí*) and GB-2 (*tīng huì*), and LR-3 (*tài chōng*). These points drain the liver and gallbladder ministerial fire and clear the heart and spirit, while quieting the orifices of the ears and eyes.

COMMENT

Electroacupuncture has a good result for excited and agitated patients. Generally, one can select one or two pairs of points and use a continuous wave with moderate strength stimulation, adjusted to patient tolerance. For a female patient with menses at the time of treatment, CV-3 (*zhōng jí*), M-CA-18 (*zǐ gōng*)[4]—three *cùn* lateral to CV-3 (*zhōng jí*), and SP-6 (*sān yīn jiāo*) may be added to regulate and rectify menstruation. A close relationship between the development of menstrual irregularity and mental diseases is frequently seen in clinical practice. If a schizophrenia patient's menstrual symptoms make a positive change, it frequently denotes a positive change in her entire condition.

4. IMPROVING THERAPEUTIC EFFECTIVENESS

Acupuncture and moxibustion have a very good effect in the treatment of schizophrenia, obtaining rewarding results particularly

---

[4]Translator's note—The name *zǐ gōng* is the common word for uterus.

with conditions that are diagnosed in the early stages. However, if a case has already surpassed one year in duration, effective treatment is then more difficult to achieve. [We would like] to point out how to improve the usual therapeutic effectiveness of acupuncture on schizophrenic disorders. Beyond accurately identifying the pattern of disease and selecting effective points, one should also master the needling sensation of directing qi below the needle, as well as gain proficiency in needle manipulation techniques for supplementing and draining.[5]

A. MASTERY OF DIRECTING QI BELOW THE NEEDLE

Acupuncture is an important part of China's traditional medicine. Its inherent special nature was developed over a long history of medical practice. When inserting needles to treat disease, the foremost task is to manipulate qi in order to course and free the channels and vessels, to harmonize qi and blood. Consequently, ancient and modern acupuncture scholars all place great importance on manipulation techniques. They all emphasize mastering the movement of qi below the needle (i.e., "needle sensation" as referred to hereinafter).

Within the human body, qi is the most basic, fundamental component of essential substance and of all complex functions. It circulates cyclically, maintains normal biological functions of the human body, and plays a role of utmost importance within all life activities.

Thus, as the *Nán Jīng, "Eighth Difficulty"* points out, "Qi is the basic root of a person." Qi has the function of resisting evils; thus it is called "correct qi." The ancients used a variety of names to refer to correct qi, such as "true qi," "original qi," "spirit qi," "yang qi," and "channel qi." Zhāng Jǐng Yuè of the Ming Dynasty said, "Correct qi is also called spirit qi." *Elementary Questions, "Lǐ Hé Zhēn Xié Lùn"* says, "True qi is channel qi."

---

[5]Translator's note—It is said that an acupuncturist's ability can be assessed by judging three skills: pattern identification, point selection, and manipulation techniques. The authors' comments here make reference to these skills.

Qi is the content of channels, network vessels, and acupuncture points. Acupuncture points are spread over the surface of the body where the channels and network vessels circulate and communicate. Thus they are also called "channel points." They are the places on the body surface where the qi of the channels, network vessels, viscera, and bowels collect and gather. Needling is one method for manipulating the body's correct qi or channel qi to cure disease. *Líng Shū, "Xié Kè"* says:

Freeing the paths and eliminating evils [using the channel points] supplements insufficiencies, drains superabundances, and regulates vacuity and repletion.

When performing acupuncture, the ancients took very seriously "the dynamic within the empty," the needle sensation within acupuncture points. They emphasized that good acupuncture requires skill at controlling the qi below the needle, and clinical experience shows that the quality of an acupuncturist's manipulation methods is primarily determined by the degree to which he or she can control channel qi. Mastering needle sensation to the extent that one can make the qi arrive at the location of disease is the crucial challenge for improving clinical effectiveness in acupuncture.

For example, PC-6 *(nèi guān)* can treat diseases of the heart, liver, stomach, and other viscera. The poem *Wǔ Zǒng Xué Gē* says, "Plot PC-6 *(nèi guān)* for the chest and lateral costal regions." If one can direct the qi below the needle to move to the elbow, to the brachium, and to arrive at the axillary-thoracic region, an immediate effect will usually be had on pain of the heart, stomach, or liver viscera, and even on auricular fibrillation.

Applying masterful techniques for manipulating qi below the needle and making it arrive at the place of disease is also an important subject in *Líng Shū, "Cì Jiē Zhēn Xié Lùn"*:

When employing the varieties of needling, [the gist] is in regulating qi.

Huá Tuó, the famous Han Dynasty physician, had abundant clinical experience in this regard. [He wrote]:

If needling a patient, use not more than one or two points. When the needle is inserted, explain what you anticipate will result; when [the qi] is about to arrive, say something to the patient. When the patient acknowledges [the sensation], the qi has arrived. The needle should then be removed and the disease will be cured.

We can observe that in addition to very highly developed needling technique, Huá Tuó not only was familiar with the position and movement of qi (*"what you anticipate will result"*), he could also sense via the sensation in his fingers where the qi had reached, and could communicate it to patients (*when [the qi] is about to arrive, say something to the patient"*). Relying on such a high level of acupuncture skill, on the occasion that "Cáo Cāo was plagued with accumulated suffering and head wind with dizziness," when "Huá Tuó's hand did simple needling the disease was cured."

Mastery in guiding the qi below the needle does not occur naturally merely by hearing of it, nor does it happen by chance. It is decided by the skill in the physician's technique.

Our clinical experience in striving for the ability to manipulate qi and make it radiate to the location of disease has shown that one must do more than attain proficiency in the basic needle manipulations. One should also be thoroughly familiar with three essential subjects: point location, direction of the needle, and depth of insertion. When [understanding of] these three essential subjects is combined with frequent clinical practice, one can be a proficient and versatile health-care provider.

POINT LOCATION

This refers to finding the precise location of an acupuncture point. Different writings from the ancient dynasties frequently have contradictory descriptions regarding how to locate particular points. Let us examine GB-20 (*fēng chí*) as an example of a commonly used point. The Wang edition of *Elementary Questions*, "*Qì Fǔ Lùn*" says:

[Fēng chí is located] in the depression posterior to the ear; when pressure is applied, it causes a response in the ear.

The *Jiǎ Yī Jīng* affirms:

[*Fēng chí* is located] posterior to the temple, in the depression along the hairline.

The *Zī Shēng Jīng* describes it thus:

[*Fēng chí* is located] posterior to GB-19 (nǎo kōng) in the depression along the hairline.

The *Míng Táng* gives this location:

[*Fēng chí*] is level with GV-16 (fēng fǔ), located exactly two cùn lateral from it.

In the *Lèi Jīng Tú Yì*, its position is recorded [in the following manner]:

[*Fēng chí* is] posterior to the ear and posterior to the temple, below nǎo kōng (GB-19) within the depression on the hairline. When pressure is applied it causes a response in the ear.

The *Jīng Xué Zuǎn Yào* describes its location as follows:

[*Fēng chí* is] the point between TB-16 (tiān yǒu) and BL-10 (tiān zhù).

The *Shù Xué Zhé Zhōng* gives its location as follows:

[*Fēng chí* is] to the side of GV-15 (yǎ mén), straight on the hairline.

The *Zhēn Jiǔ Dà Chéng* and the *Zhēn Jiǔ Jù Yīng* record this location:

[*Fēng chí* is] posterior to the ear, and posterior to the temple, below nǎo kōng (GB-19) in the depression along the hairline. When pressure is applied there is a response in the ear.

Further examples abound. With such a diversity of conflicting advice, one cannot decide upon any single point. Our own experience has shown that GB-20 (fēng chí) should be precisely located level with the earlobe, within the depression on the hairline (similar to the *míng táng* location). If we consider that certain points have over ten differing point locations, and if we ponder how this came to be, [we can surmise that] perhaps it was due to poor or unsystematic knowledge of anatomy in the ancient dynasties. This may have led to sketchiness in ancient recordings, and individual differences in the experiences of acupuncturists. To be successful in clinical practice, precise locations must be known for each point selected.

PROPER DIRECTION OF NEEDLING

The phrase "direction of needling" bears no association to descriptions in common acupuncture texts regarding the angle of needle insertion. This is because the angle of insertion is usually decided by the thickness of muscle at the body surface. For example, when needling the scalp or face, in the regions of scant flesh, one usually uses an oblique or transverse insertion angle. In regions of the body where muscle is thick, perpendicular insertions are used. The "direction of needling" to which we refer in this context means the precise direction of the needle as it penetrates the surface and causes movement of qi to distal parts.

For directional positioning, each point is unique, yet each point has corresponding [marks that] fix its individual positioning. Using the example of GB-20 (*fēng chí*) again, and locating it level with the ear lobe at the inferior margin of the hairline, the needle should be gradually inserted and the needle tip should be guided in a criss-crossing pattern directed toward the inferior margin of the cheekbone, such that when needling GB-20 (*fēng chí*) on the patient's left side, the needle tip is directed toward the inferior margin of the right cheekbone. When needling GB-20 (*fēng chí*) on the right side, the tip of the needle is directed toward the inferior margin of the left cheekbone.

If in addition one masters the exact depth of insertion, normally the qi under the needle can be propagated from the anterior region of the brain to the forehead or eye region. Otherwise, the needle sensation usually is limited to the local region of the needle, and does not reach distant points.

PROPER DEPTH OF NEEDLE INSERTION

In the ancient acupuncture writings, the rules for depth of needle insertion mostly specified more shallow insertion than what is clinically practical. Perhaps this was careful prudence on behalf of the ancient physicians who held serious concerns about needling too deeply into important viscera or blood vessels. Thus, they encouraged the safety of more shallow needling over the risk of deeper needling. As a result, if one needles according to their instructions, it is often impossible to get the qi to radiate to distant points. In the example of GB-20 *(fēng chí)* given above, most writings suggest a depth of only 3-4 *fēn*.[6]

Clinical practice proves that a depth of 1-1.5 *cùn* is necessary on this point for qi from the posterior brain and temporal regions to radiate to the forehead and eye regions. If one directs the needle toward the GB-20 *(fēng chí)* point on the opposite side, the needle sensation can circulate down from the cervical spinal region.

The three essential topics explained above must be construed as interrelated. For example, if the needle has already reached a certain depth and there is still no radiation of needle sensation, one should reconsider the accuracy of the point location as well as the direction of the needle in order to avoid creating accidents by blindly needling too deeply.

B. PROPER APPLICATION OF SUPPLEMENTING AND DRAINING METHODS

Correctly applying supplementing and draining manipulations is another critical skill for effective acupuncture. We consider acupuncture to be an informational therapy that applies external forces. Through this informational input, it relies on an organism's natural curative capacities to internally recover harmony of yin and yang. Acupuncture and medicinal therapies are most definitely different. Every medicinal formula has certain principles of combination and parameters of use.

───

[6]Translator's note—A *fēn* is the Chinese medical measure for 1/10th of a *cùn* or body inch. The width of a patient's four fingers equals three body inches for that patient.

For example, any common formula that frees the stool is not able to check diarrhea. Formulas that check diarrhea are likewise unable to free the stool. However, when acupuncture treats two opposite diseases that affect one viscus (such as constipation and diarrhea), frequently the same points are chosen and the only difference is whether the manipulation technique supplements or drains. This is observed repeatedly in the acupuncture literature of dynasty after dynasty.

For example, *Lán Jiāng Fǔ* states:

> *For damaging cold with absence of sweating, drain LI-4 (hé gǔ) and supplement KI-7 (fù liū). If there is copious persistent perspiration, supplement LI-4 (hé gǔ) and drain KI-7 (fù liū).*

Zhēn Jiǔ Dà Chéng records:

> *Wén Bó drains SP-6 (sān yīn jiāo) and supplements LI-4 (hé gǔ); the fetus responds to the acupuncture and descends.*

> *Now, we cannot supplement SP-6 (sān yīn jiāo) and drain LI-4 (hé gǔ) to quiet the fetus. In short, SP-6 (sān yīn jiāo) is the intersection point of the kidney, liver, and spleen vessels; it governs yin and blood, and should be supplemented, not drained. LI-4 (hé gǔ) is the source point of the large intestine channel; the large intestine is the bowel associated with the lungs, and governing qi. It should be drained and not supplemented.*

These examples illuminate that when using the same combination of points, merely employing different supplementing and draining manipulations, [produces] effects that are completely opposite. Thus, *Qiān Jīn Fāng* records the saying:

> *When using the method of needling, emphasize supplementing and draining.*

The following manipulations are some of the acupuncture supplementing and draining techniques that are commonly used in modern times. They include methods such as lifting and thrusting for supplementing and draining, rotational supplementing and draining, and even supplementing–even draining. They are a simple introduction to the authors' findings.

C. LIFTING AND THRUSTING FOR SUPPLEMENTING AND DRAINING

CONCEPTUAL BASIS

According to the foundational concepts of yin and yang natures, the surface of the body ascribes to yang, and the interior of the body ascribes to yin. The *Zhēn Jiǔ Dà Chéng* says:

> When one is draining, first go deep and later shallow; from inside induce a hold and let it out. When one is supplementing, first go shallow and later deep; from the outside push to the inside and make [qi] enter. It is because of how yin and yang relate to inside and outside that the needle is inserted and withdrawn.

[With this method] one adjusts the body's qi in its constructive, defensive, internal, external, yin, and yang aspects, and thereby the body can be restored to a balance of yin and yang.

SCOPE OF APPLICATION

This method is mostly employed when needling visceral and bowel points on the body's trunk. Besides being suited to the conceptual basis of this method, it also does not cause injuries if one mistakenly needles into an organ (i.e., if the liver were punctured with this manipulation there would be no damaging rotational movement).

MANIPULATION

The *Nán Jīng*, "Seventy-Eighth Difficulty," states:

> Obtaining qi and pushing it inward is called supplementation; moving and extending it is called draining.

Furthermore, all the Ming Dynasty schools had admonitions such as:

> Quickly lift and slowly press ... it is draining. Slowly lift and quickly press ... it is supplementing.

This means that once the needle has been inserted and the qi has been obtained, the needle is moved up and down with lifting and thrusting, first at a shallow level, afterwards at the deeper levels. Repetitions with heavy thrusting and light lifting (rapid pressing and slow lifting) is considered supplementation. In contrast, using repetitions of heavy lifting and light thrusting (rapid lifting and slow thrusting) that begin in the deeper levels and later [are done] in the shallow levels, is considered draining.

Mania disease type is ascribed to yang and is generally repletion. Thus, when needling surface points of the viscera and bowels on the trunk, it is usually suitable to employ a lifting and thrusting draining method.

D. ROTATIONAL SUPPLEMENTING–DRAINING METHOD

Conceptual Basis

Zhēn Jiŭ Dà Chéng records:

> *When talking of constructive and defensive qi, they are where the internal and external enter and exit. When discussing the channels and vessels, they are where the qi comes and goes up and down. For each of these one goes to the place where qi resides, and needles to normalize counterflow.*

The lifting and thrusting, supplementing–draining method explained above depends on harmonizing the entering and exiting of constructive and defensive qi from inside to outside. The latter method, or rotational supplementing–draining method, has the purpose of harmonizing the upward and downward coming and going of qi in the channels and vessels. Thus the basis of the rotational supplementing–draining method is the promotion of free qi and blood flow in the channels and vessels.

Scope of Application

Drawing from this conceptual basis, one usually employs rotational supplementing–draining manipulation when points are selected from the four limbs.

Manipulation

According to *Shén Zhēn Bā Fǎ:*

> *When one is draining there is the phoenix spreading its wings. Use the index finger and thumb of the right hand to grasp the head of the needle, and, like an image of soaring, grasp and release [the needle]. ... When one is supplementing there is the hungry horse ringing the bell. Use the index finger and thumb of the right hand to grasp the head of the needle. As if a hungry horse with no strength, move it in very slowly, and then later withdraw it quickly.*

In this manipulation, after inserting the needle and obtaining qi, rotating heavily in a large arc is a draining method. The opposite manipulation, rotating relatively lightly in a relatively small arc, is a supplementing method.

Mania disease type is ascribed to yang and is generally repletion. Thus, when needling points of the four limbs, it is usually suitable to employ rotational draining method.

E. EVEN SUPPLEMENTING—EVEN DRAINING METHOD

Conceptual Basis

Líng Shū, "*Wǔ Luàn*" says:

> *Slowly inserting and slowly withdrawing is called conducting qi. It conforms to neither supplementing nor draining, and is called the "same essence." There is no superabundance or insufficiency; chaotic qi is in counterflow.*

In this method one abducts and outthrusts evil qi to the outside, and directs correct qi for recovery. Such is the basis of this method for summoning qi.

Scope of Application

From the concept explained above ("There is no superabundance or insufficiency; chaotic qi is in counterflow"), [we can see that] this method is suitable for cases where neither vacuity nor repletion is particularly apparent, or cases where there is both vacuity and repletion, as well as for diseases where the body temporarily has chaotic qi and blood.

MANIPULATION TECHNIQUE

After inserting the needle and obtaining qi, administer even lifting and thrusting, and a rotation of the needle that is neither slow nor fast. Gauge the appropriate needle sensation by what the patient can tolerate. After rotating the needle for a few minutes, withdraw it.

The withdrawal disease type is ascribed to yin and is generally vacuity with repletion complication. Thus, this method is often used to support the correct and dispel evils to simultaneously supplement and drain.

II. TREATMENTS BASED ON ANCIENT EXPERIENCES

Chinese medical sciences have a long history. As early as the *Líng Shū* there was a thorough description of mania-withdrawal and its treatment. In addition, there have been many accounts scattered within other writings. For example, regarding "yang reversal" angered mania patients, *Elementary Questions, "Bìng Néng Lùn"* advocates treatment either by fasting or by ingesting crude iron flakes (*shēng tiě luò*). The *Líng Shū* is predominantly about acupuncture and moxibustion, and it contains abundant information that suggests various regions to needle for a variety of symptoms. Since the *Líng Shū* there have been numerous accounts in the medical writings of every dynasty. The important ones are discussed below.

1. CLASSICAL ACUPUNCTURE THERAPY FOR TREATMENT OF MANIA DISEASE

In *Líng Shū*, *"Diān Kuáng"* it is recorded:

> When mania (*kuáng*) arises, [the patient takes] scant rest and [has] no hunger. There are self-delusions of superiority and virtuousness, of discernment and wisdom, of honor and respectability;

[such patients are] given to cursing day and night. To treat, select hand yáng míng, tài yáng, and tài yīn, under[-side of] the tongue, and shào yin. Seeing the case in exuberance, employ all points. If not in exuberance, then reduce suitably.

We interpret this passage of classical Chinese to say that when patients start to have mania they generally have no desire to sleep, and do not feel hunger. They consider themselves incomparable—supremely intelligent, honorable, and respectable —and will have other manifestations of abnormal intellect. It is common for them to see someone and immediately begin cussing. Day and night, they are incessantly boisterous.

For acupuncture treatment, one should select points from the hand *yáng míng* large intestine channel, the hand *tài yáng* small intestine channel, and the hand *tài yīn* lung channel, as well as the subglossal points and the hand *shào yīn* heart channel. In the Ming Dynasty, Mǎ Yuán Tái held that the actual points were: LI-6 (*piān lì*), LI-7 (*wēn liù*), SI-7 (*zhī zhèng*), SI-8 (*xiǎo hǎi*), LU-7 (*liè què*), and LU-9 (*tài yuān*), as well as the subglossal point CV-23 (*lián quán*), and points HT-7 (*shén mén*) and HT-9 (*shào chōng*) of the hand *shào yīn* heart channel.

If the case is critical, use all these channel points. If the disease is not severe, one should select a few of the points on the basis of circumstances. Editors in subsequent dynasties commonly accepted Mǎ Yuán Tái's interpretation. However, in present times it is rare for anyone to use these points when treating mania.

Zhēn Jiǔ Jiǎ Yǐ Jīng [contains comments such as]:

For mania with copious, unceasing speech and crazed running (about), a desire to commit suicide, and confused vision, needle GV-16 (fēng fǔ).

Tendency to mania is governed by LU-10 (yú jì), LI-4 (hé gǔ), SI-4 (wán gǔ), SI-7 (zhī zhèng), HT-3 (shào hǎi), and BL-60 (kūn lún).[7]

---

[7]Translator's note—In this section, the word "govern" connotes that the points mentioned govern the treatment of the symptoms indicated.

For manic raving, LU-9 (tài yuān) governs.

For mania, TB-2 (yè mén) governs.

For mania, TB-2 (yè mén) governs, as do GB-42 (jiā xī), GB-40 (qiū xū), and GB-37 (guāng míng).

For mania and withdrawal, KI-10 (yīn gŭ) governs.

For mania with running about and frequent yawning, ST-37 (jù xū) and LI-9 (shàng lián) govern.[8]

For mania with visions of ghosts and fires, ST-41 (jiĕ xī) governs.

Zhēn Jiŭ Zī Shēng Jīng [contains statements such as]:

GV-16 (fēng fŭ) and BL-13 (fèi shū) govern manic walking and temptation to suicide.

ST-42 (chōng yáng) and ST-40 (fēng lóng) govern mania with desire for climbing to a high place and singing out, or throwing off clothes and running amok.

BL-10 (tiān zhù) and GB-41(zú lín qī)[9] *govern mania tendencies with ceaseless talkativeness and upturned eyes.*

SI-7 (zhī zhèng), LU-10 (yú jì), LI-4 (hé gŭ), HT-3 (shào hăi), LI-11 (qū chí), and SI-4 (wán gŭ) govern manic raving.

LI-8 (xià lián) and GB-40 (quī xū) govern extraordinarily manic speech.

CV-14 (jù què) and KI-9 (zhú bīn) govern mania and raving with angered cussing.

GV-16 (fēng fŭ) treats manic running (about) with a desire for suicide, and upturned eyes with confused vision.

ST-42 (chōng yáng) treats chronic mania with climbing to high places and singing, throwing off clothes and running amok.

GB-37 (guāng míng) treats sudden onset mania.

SI-5 (yáng gŭ) treats withdrawal disease with manic running [about].

GV-14 (jù què) treats mania with failure to recognize people and fright palpitations with shortage of qi.

---

[8]Translator's note—*Jù xū* could mean either ST-37 or ST-39 .

[9]Translator's note—*Lín qī* could mean either GB-41 *zú lín qī* or GB-15 *(tóu lín qī)*.

Zhēn Jiŭ Dà Chéng, "*Xīn Xié Diān Kuáng Mén*" states:

> *Mania-withdrawal:* LI-11 (*qū chí*), SI-8 (*xiăo hăi*), HT-3 (*shào hăi*), PC-5 (*jiān shĭ*), LI-5 (*yáng xī*), SI-5 (*yáng gŭ*), PC-7 (*dà líng*), LI-4 (*hé gŭ*), LU-10 (*yú jì*), SI-4 (*wán gŭ*), HT-7 (*shén mén*), TB-2 (*yè mén*), ST-42 (*chōng yáng*), LR-2 (*xíng jiān*), BL-64 (*jīng gŭ*), BL-13 (*fèi shū*) [*and other points*].

The points recorded in the ancient selections above are still employed today, and have definite therapeutic effects.

2. CLASSICAL ACUPUNCTURE THERAPY FOR WITHDRAWAL (*DIĀN*) DISEASE TYPE

Líng Shū, "*Diān Kuáng*" states:

> *When withdrawal begins, at first [the patient is] unhappy, [has a] heavy head and aches, [as well as] staring vision and red eyes. A more extreme development is vexation of the heart. Diagnose by the color. Select the hand tài yáng, hand yáng míng, and hand tài yīn. When the blood changes, that is the end.*

We interpret this as saying that at the onset of this disease, the patient will first feel depressed and unhappy, with a heavy feeling in the head and headaches. Both eyes stare straight ahead, and are reddened. At the next more serious step of development there can be heart vexation, agitation, and unquieted emotions. When diagnosing this illness, one may observe the hue of the Celestial Court (*tiān tíng*) [in the center of the forehead].

For treatment, one may select hand *tài yáng* small intestine channel points SI-7 (*zhī zhèng*) and SI-8 (*xiăo hăi*), hand *yáng míng* large intestine points LI-6 (*piān lì*) and LI-7 (*wēn liù*), and as well hand *tài yīn* lung channel points LU-7 (*liè quē*), and LU-9 (*tài yuān*). We can see that except for the three points CV-23 (*lián quán*), HT-7 (*shén mén*), and HT-9 (*shào chōng*), the points selected are the same as the points that treat mania.

It is worth noting that before the Ming Dynasty, despite an abundance of accounts with constantly increasing differentiations of schizophrenia, the perceptions of withdrawal (*diān*) and epilepsy *(xián)* were still intertwined and indistinct. The two characters *diān* and *xián* were used interchangeably. As an example, in *Zhū Bìng Yuán Hòu Lún,* Cháo Yuán Fāng stated:

> *When over age ten, it is withdrawal (diān); when under age ten, it is epilepsy (xián).*

In fact these both refer to epileptic mal.

Furthermore, during the Tang Dynasty, Sūn Sī Miǎo, writing in *Qiān Jīn Fāng,* pointed out five kinds of withdrawal diseases; from the symptoms described they are mostly epileptic seizures. For example, in "yáng withdrawal," "at the onset [the patient] looks as if dead, and has enuresis, [then] is resolved in a moment." This is to say that the patient suddenly loses consciousness and involuntarily discharges urine, and in a moment the episode is over.

This [lack of distinction between disease types] prevailed until the Ming Dynasty when Wáng Kěn Táng wrote *Zhèng Zhì Zhǔn Shéng.* This work provided a systematic summary of all mental disorders, thus forming a relatively complete specialty in mental disorders. The two diseases of withdrawal *(diān)* and epilepsy *(xián)* were clearly distinguished, reforming the confusion of categorizations in mental disorder types. Wáng Kěn Táng thus became the father of all later mania–withdrawal studies. Thus the historical context should be remembered when studying ancient texts.

> *Zhēn Jiǔ Jiǎ Yǐ Jīng* states:
>
> *[For] withdrawal accompanied by anger and desire to murder, GV-12 (shēn zhù) governs.*
>
> *For withdrawal, BL-17 (gé shū) and BL-18 (gān shū) govern.*
>
> *For sighing and proclivity to sorrow, for fever in the lower abdomen and desire to go about, GB-24 (rì yuè) governs.*
>
> *For manic raving, LU-9 (tài yuān) governs.*
>
> *When the heart feels anxious and empty, and the patient has a hungry appearance, with tendency to sorrow along with frightmania, red face, and yellow eyes, PC-5 (jiān shǐ) governs.*
>
> *For mania and withdrawal, SI-5 (yáng gǔ), KI-9 (zhú bīn), and BL-66 (tōng gǔ) govern.*

For withdrawal and mania, often with overpowering inclinations to eat and to laugh but not show it outwardly, and with vexation and thirst, SP-5 (shāng qiū) governs.

Zhēn Jiǔ Zī Shēng Jīng records [comments such as]:

HT-7 (shén mén) and SI-5 (yáng gǔ) govern laughing as if manic.

PC-8 (láo gōng) and PC-7 (dà líng) govern wind heat with a tendency to anger, joy and sorrow in the heart, wanting to cry yet actually laughing, and ceaseless laughter.

LI-7 (wēn liù) and BL-61 (pú cān) govern withdrawal, protrusion of the tongue and swelling of the chin, raving, and seeing ghosts.

PC-5 (jiān shǐ) governs fright mania with a tendency to sorrow, red face and yellow eyes, loss of speech.

SI-5 (yáng gǔ), GV-12 (shēn zhù), GB-19 (nǎo kōng), and BL-64 (jīng gǔ) treat withdrawal with running amok.

BL-65 (shù gǔ) treats mania-withdrawal.

HT-7 (shén mén) treats generalized fever and manic sorrow with crying.

PC-7 (dà líng) treats manic raving and unhappiness.

LI-6 (piān lì) treats withdrawal with copious speech.

LI-8 (xià lián) treats manic raving.

Zhēn Jiǔ Dà Chéng, "Xīn Xié Diān Kuáng Mén" [includes comments such as]:

For withdrawal: GV-23 (shàng xīng), GV-20 (bǎi huì), GB-20 (fēng chí), LI-11 (qū chí), LU-5 (chǐ zé), LI-5 (yáng xī), SI-4 (wán gǔ), ST-41 (jiě xī), SI-3 (hòu xī), BL-62 (shēn mài), BL-60 (kūn lún), SP-5 (shāng qiū), KI-2 (rán gǔ), BL-66 (tōng gǔ), BL-57 (chéng shān).

All points mentioned above are still used in the modern clinic within combinations for specific circumstances.

In addition to these writings, there are many rhymes and verses penned by acupuncture authors that record how to treat mania and withdrawal. For example, Tōng Xuán Zhǐ Yào Fù has:

HT-7 (*shén mén*) *eliminates feeble-mindedness [related to the heart].* ... *For epilepsy fits with withdrawal and mania, rely on SI-3 (hòu xī) for a rectifying cure.*

Líng Guāng Fù records:

GV-26 (*shuǐ gōu*) *and PC-5 (jiān shǐ) treat evil withdrawal.*

Xí Hóng Fù records:

GV-26 (*rén zhōng*) *treats withdrawal with great efficacy; the thirteen ghost points are not necessary.*

Yù Lóng Fù records:

HT-7 (*shén mén*) *treats feeble-mindedness with laughing and sobbing.*

Yù Lóng Gē records:

For feeble-mindedness with aversion to proximity of family [and] indiscriminately reviling people regardless of their social status, HT-7 (*shén mén*) *alone cures feeble-mindedness; turn the hand to spread the bones and get the true point.*

These songs and poems are mostly summaries of our ancestors' clinical experience. The words are simple, the meanings concise. They comprise one portion of a valuable legacy within the treasure chest of acupuncture.

The *Líng Shū* records the following within two sections, "*Jīng Mài*," and "*Jiǔ Zhēn Shí Èr Yuán*":

When there is exuberance, drain it; when there is vacuity, supplement it. For heat, treat rapidly; for cold, retain. For falling downward, use moxibustion; for neither exuberance nor vacuity, use the channel to grasp it.

What was lush and then clogged, eliminate.

These [early comments] formed the principles of therapy for acupuncture pattern identification, and supplementing–draining needling. This means that acupuncture and moxibustion therapy, built upon the foundation of channel theory, included the methods of "identifying patterns of vacuity and repletion, and applying treatments to supplement and drain." Thus, acupuncturists in the ancient dynasties not only emphasized accurate pattern identification and suitable point selection, they also valued the use of needle manipulations for supplementation and draining. *Líng Shū, "Xié Qì Zàng Fǔ Bìng Xíng"* states:

> *If supplementing and draining are reversed, the diseases can become critical.*

Undoubtedly, this topic also deserves research within the study of mania-withdrawal acupuncture treatments.

3. OTHER ANCIENT MEASURES

From their extensive clinical practice the doctors of antiquity accumulated abundant experience in treating schizophrenic disorders. They were greatly concerned about the significance of emotional disharmony as a contributing factor to the onset of a disease. Not only did the physicians of antiquity use acupuncture, moxibustion, and medicinal agents to treat patients, they also emphasized psychological therapies and sleep therapy. We believe that this is one of the greatest contributions to Chinese medical history. The saying attributed to ancient Persian medical scholars, "Physicians have three weapons with which to treat disease: talk, herbs [medicines], and knives," quite coincidentally also represents this notion.

A. MENTAL THERAPY (PSYCHOLOGICAL THERAPY)

Elementary Questions, "Bǎo Mìng Quán Xíng Lùn" records that "therapy of the spirit" is among the five methods of therapy. It emphasizes that "one must first treat the spirit," which is noted to mean to adjust and treat the essence-spirit, and focus treatment on [the patient's] heart.

This is mental therapy that does not involve acupuncture or medicinal agents. Ancient scholars felt that in treating patients, winning trust and confidence was an important prerequisite. They emphasized the mental therapies of instructing, guiding, and opening as treatments for disease, and pointed out that an important aspect of treatment is to apply therapy for the seven affects [psychological therapy] to assist acupuncture and medicinal agents.

For example, we read in the *Líng Shū*, *"Shī Fù"*:

Huáng Dì said: "[Regarding the diet of] those wealthy people who eat rich, fatty foods, who show no restraint in giving in to pleasures, and who make light of people who advise them to change their ways, for [a doctor] to stop them would oppose their will; yet to go along with them would allow their illnesses to get worse. How should such patients be dealt with? What should be treated first?"

Qí Bó said: "The emotions of humans are such that everyone has an aversion to death and a love for life. You [should] explain to them how they are failing, tell them what is good, lead them to the correct course, and open their eyes to their suffering. Although there are people who do not have an understanding of these things, who would not comply?"

We can see that as early as two thousand years ago, Chinese physicians endorsed giving explanations, comfort, and guidance when treating patients.

The development of "adjusting" therapies in the Jin-Yuan period was the practical application of psychotherapeutic methods.[10] The representative physicians were Zhāng Zǐ Hé—one of the four great physicians of the Jin-Yuan period—and the renowned physician-scholar of the Ming Dynasty, Zhāng Jīng Yuè. The next section introduces and explains a few pertinent examples from ancient case histories.

---

[10]Translator's note: Numerous experts were baffled by the characters that are translated here as "adjusting." The characters are pronounced *huó tào* and have the literal meaning of "slipknot." One explanation was that it referred to the adjustable nature of determining treatments on the basis of the pattern of disease, thus the translation offered here. However, no one else recognized these characters in this way. Perhaps it is a misprint in the text.

A CASE BY ZHĀNG ZǏ HÉ

(FROM "COMMENTARIES ON ANCIENT AND MODERN MEDICAL CASE
HISTORIES," BY YÚ ZHÈN, QING DYNASTY)

A lady had hunger but no desire to eat. Moreover, she was
not happy, and at times she cussed and cursed. Extensive
treatment was ineffective. Zhāng Dài Rén (Zhāng Zǐ Hé)
reviewed the case and said, "This is difficult to treat with
medicines." So he had two women put on makeup and play
as actresses.

The lady was very amused. The following day he had the
two women play roles again, which again made the lady
very happy. Then he made everyone around eat beside her
and praise the delicious food. The lady was moved and also
ate a little. She was advised to avoid partaking excessively.
After several days, the disease had declined and the lady's
appetite had increased. She was fully cured.

COMMENT

This disease was from anxiety and thought damaging the spleen,
and applies to illness resulting from psychological causes. *Líng
Shū*, "*Běn Shén*" states:

> When the spleen has unresolved worry and anxiety, then [the
> ability to] reflect is damaged. When reflection is damaged then
> there is chaos.

> In those with worry and anxiety, the qi is blocked and does not
> move.

Due to the qi binding and damaging the spleen, movement
and transformation are impaired. Thus, in this disease there is
hunger with no desire to eat, and reflection is damaged and
chaotic. Spleen qi binds and then rebels against liver-wood; this
represses and depresses liver qi. At times there is cussing and
cursing, which signifies that depressed wood desires outthrust.

When *Elementary Questions,* "*Xuān Míng Wǔ Qì*" states, "the
liver['s illness] is speech," it refers to precisely this instance. As

the disease was from anxiety and [excessive] thought, the first necessity was to eliminate the psychological disharmony.

Zhāng Zǐ Hé relied on the reasoning that joy prevails over anxiety, as stated in *Elementary Questions*. He first made the lady happy in order to forget her anxieties and to harmonize her mind. Next he made her see the tasty foods, to inspire her appetite. Because his treatment and guidance were methodical, the patient was cured within a few days but did not require medicinal agents.

MEDICAL CASE HISTORY OF WÁNG ZHŌNG YÁNG

(FROM GǓ JĪN MÍNG YĪ LÈI ÁN, BY JIĀNG GUÀN, MING DYNASTY)

One lady suspected her husband had a lover, and became sick with loss of heart and confusion. She talked ceaselessly through the day and night, and kept patrolling around her home, [but was] unable to catch anyone.

Dr. Wang administered 80 Phlegm-Rolling Pills (*Gǔn Tán Wán*). She immediately pretended to sleep and for that night she did not speak. The second night another batch was given. Altogether she had two doses, and expelled some [fecal] matter.

The patient felt ashamed, and began to eat and sit up as normal. After five to seven days she could do needlework, but in the end she could not get free from the idea [that her husband had a lover].

Wang pondered the relapse and secretly ordered someone to go before the patient and announce to another person at her side, "What a pity that such and such a woman suddenly died of summerheat stroke."

The patient was elated! She asked: "How do you know that?"

The speaker said: "I have seen her husband preparing the funeral." The patient had a joyful radiance and from that moment gradually recovered.

COMMENT

In the *Lei Jing*, Zhāng Jǐng Yuè also cited this case when explaining *Elementary Questions*, "*Yí Jīng Biàn Qì Lùn.*" Zhāng Jǐng Yuè states:

> *The seven affects in humans are engendered by their likes and dislikes. When likes and dislikes grow out of proportion, then qi tends to gather. With tendency to gather then there is surfeit and deficit, and the spirit-mind is easily chaotic. When the spirit-mind has [deviated] tendencies, and evils repeatedly reside there, then ghosts arise in the heart. Thus, when someone has many dislikes, they see what is unlikable.*

"Ghosts arise in the heart" connotes the patient's abnormal psychology. In this example it means the jealousy and suspicions in the patient's heart. For patients with diseases that originate from jealousy, one can use a method to shift essence and change qi to remove the dislikes. In this case, because the patient suspected her husband had a lover, she lost heart and developed manic confusion.

The excellence of Wáng Zhōng Yáng's treatment method was that he did not use a heart-settling, spirit-quieting formula, nor did he explain the problem to her husband. Instead, he used the psychological method of "removing what is disliked." He had someone give the false message that her husband's lover had suddenly died of summerheat stroke. Thus, when the patient heard the news she was happy and her face had a joyful radiance. "Heart diseases" can be seen to naturally subside like this.

This example illustrates that when treating schizophrenic patients one must be competent at grasping the pattern of their psychological activities. There are times when the skillful use of speech with the precision of an archer is an extraordinary necessity for the sake of guiding patients.

A MEDICAL CASE HISTORY BY XÚ HUÍ XĪ

(FROM MEDICAL CASE HISTORIES BY XÚ HUÍ XĪ, QING DYNASTY.)

The Diàn Zhuàn scholar had recently tested out as the top scholar in the imperial examinations. He took a leave of absence to return home, and upon arriving at Zhǔn had taken ill.

He sought a famous physician. The doctor said: "This illness cannot be treated. In seven days you will die. You should go home quickly; perhaps you can reach there in time."

The Diàn Zhuàn scholar became gloomy and despondent, and set about his journey with all due haste. After seven days had passed there was no illness.

His servant stepped forward and said, "The doctor had a letter. He told me to present it to you when we arrived."

The Diàn Zhuàn scholar unsealed it and read: "After passing your exam great joy damaged your heart; this is not something for medicines to treat. So I mentioned dying to frighten you, as a way to cure the disease. Now there is no problem."

The Diàn Zhuàn scholar had great admiration!

COMMENT

Joyful happiness is a normal human affection. A suitable degree of joy can harmonize the emotions and free the flows and out-thrusts of constructive [qi], defensive [qi], qi, and blood. Thus, *Líng Shū, "Běn Shén"* states:

> *When the wise cultivate health ... they harmonize joy and anger and reside in quietude.*

A proverb also says: "When someone meets a joyful event, the essence-spirit flags."

Great joy in excessive measure can induce uncontrolled psychological activity which may initiate disease. This is like the statement of *Elementary Questions, "Yīn Yáng Yīng Xiàng Dà Lùn"*: "Sudden joy damages the heart." *Líng Shū, "Běn Shén"* states:

In those who are happy and joyful the spirit is frightened, dissipated, and not stored..

In this patient's case he had just placed first in the imperial examinations:

After ten years in a cold study, all at once his every move was known throughout the land.[11]

One can immediately comprehend this image of fulminant joy. It is easy to understand that the heart-spirit would fail to keep [to its abode] under the circumstances. The heart blood had been dulled and consumed, while the root of disease was concealed.

How did the famous doctor know this? Although the case history itself provides no explanation, it must have been derived from the four examinations. In this case the therapy was to treat by not treating. First, a danger warning created fear, for fear made the qi could go downward and allowed the spirit qi to return to its abode while allowing the true qi to reside within. Afterwards, the letter was sent as a reassurance, and to quiet the mind. This demonstrates the psychological therapy from *Elementary Questions,* which says that fear prevails over joy.

B. SLEEPING THERAPY

Insomnia is a common and frequent condition in the initial stages of many mental disorders. It can also worsen the state of mental disorders, or can cause a relapse. Thus, sleep is critical to mental health patients. Sleep therapy was employed very early in Chinese medical history. Sūn Sī Miǎo in the Tang Dynasty was the first to employ medicated sleeping therapy for treating mental disorders. [The following story] is recorded:

---

[11]Translator's note—Here again the author has used classical sayings that demand fuller explanation. The first saying expresses the image of a scholar who has done diligent study in austere circumstances for a prolonged period. The second saying describes a person who has suddenly become a respected celebrity. Thus it is possible to see how such a sudden sweeping change of life circumstance would precipitate a powerful emotional response.

At the Xiāng Guó Temple during the Tang Dynasty, a [Buddhist] monk named Yún Huì suffered from withdrawal disease. He had lost his heart [lost the complete use of his faculties] for half a year, and the medicines prescribed by famous doctors were of no avail. The monk had a wealthy worldly brother, Pān, who called Sūn Sī Miǎo to treat the disease.

Sūn said, "He should get to sleep tonight, and will be cured by tomorrow."

Pān said, "I'll go ahead and give him the medicine; I will never forget your kindness."

Sūn said, "If you have something salty to eat, just give him that. When he gets thirsty, come and tell me."

During the night, the monk did become thirsty. Sun went to him and straight away asked for a measure of warm wine, into which he mixed a dose of medicine and then gave it to the patient. Shortly afterward he asked for more wine, and administered another half measure. Thereupon the monk slept for two days and nights. When he awoke, he was back to normal.

Pān thanked Sūn and asked about the treatment method. Sūn said: "Most people can quiet the spirit, but cannot enable those suffering from a clouded spirit to sleep. Within the Líng Yuàn formula there is cinnabar (*zhū shā*), spiny jujube (*suān zǎo rén*), and powdered frankincense (*rǔ xiāng*), which most people are unable to use."

Another example [from the ancient literature] is Xiāo Wú Gōng who in his youth often suffered from mental diseases. He took one dose of the above formula, slept for five days, and was cured.

Later, Chén Shì Duó of the Qing Dynasty in *Shí Shì Mì Lù* also proposed a formula for naturally inducing sleep. In addition, doctors of the historical dynasties also employed verbal counselling, massage, baths, and other therapies to treat mental disorders. These precious recordings are valuable references and each one deserves further research and development.

III. TREATMENTS GATHERED FROM MODERN REPORTS

1. OVERVIEW

In recent years there have been major developments in the use of acupuncture for schizophrenia. All the historical dynasties have abundant writings on these disorders, as they are known within the parameters of the Chinese medical concept of mania-withdrawal. There was an incident in 1951 when the *People's Daily* reported Mr. Zhū Liǎn using acupuncture to cure schizophrenia. It caught the attention of the medical world, and since that time acupuncture treatment for all kinds of mental diseases has gained broad acceptance.

In the 1960's the outstanding contribution of acupuncture to the treatment of mental diseases was electroacupuncture. The application of electroconvulsive therapy (ECT) in mental wards already has several decades of history. It is still used both domestically and abroad, and is considered the most effective therapy for endogenous melancholia. However, there has been continuous dispute over stimulating wave shapes, dosages, and so forth. In Sichuan, while using electroacupuncture in standard measure for treatment of schizophrenia, they coincidentally discovered a convulsive spasm occurring that was the same as with ECT.

With further research they found that point selection and depth of needling held a significant role in this occurrence. When GB-8 (*shuài gǔ*) and GV-20 (*bǎi huì*), or GV-20 (*bǎi huì*) and M-HN-3 (*yìn táng*) are used in tandem to pass electricity (employing a common 6-12 volt battery is sufficient), this induces a convulsive spasm similar to ECT. Because the wave shape and strength are all different from what is used in traditional electric shock, the side effects are decreased.

Tests on laboratory animals showed that when the stimulation of electroacupuncture is excessive, in the end, morphological changes that may occur in the brain and internal organs are still reversible. Clearly, electroacupuncture is a wonderful improvement upon ECT. In some localities, electroacupuncture shock has already become the standard ECT. However, sometimes the flaw of half shock still occurs, and this awaits redressment.

By combining the use of certain Chinese medicinal agents with ECT, schizophrenia can be treated so that fewer side effects such as headaches will occur. Some researchers employed combined Chinese and Western medicines, or acupuncture together with medicinal agents (primarily Chinese medicinal agents), to treat 117 cases of mental disorders. They had outstanding results, and concluded that the use of Chinese medicinal agents thoroughly corrected the patients' visceral and bowel functions, while commensurately eliminating any pathological indications. The use of needle stimulation increased the resilience of the immune system and toned the regulating functions of the central nervous system. Small dosages of Western sedative drugs were administered simultaneously [to abate psychopathy]. This kind of eclectic method is safe, effective, and convenient to perform.

There are reports from practitioners who used a very slight electric current on acupuncture points to treat 204 cases of all variety of mental disorders. In a recent period their success rate reached 97.1%.

[Additionally,] insulin shock and hypoglycemia therapy both have accepted usage in the treatment of schizophrenia. However, they require the use of large dosages and prolonged treatment, and thus are expensive and labor-intensive. Furthermore, when the quantity of sugars used is relatively large, continuous dizziness is not infrequently seen. Thus, reducing dosages while reaching the therapeutic goal has been a topic of research for many years.

The clinical trials mentioned below used small doses injected at acupuncture points, in combination with weak electronic stimulation on the points, to produce satisfactory results that were equal to standard therapy in effect but far more cost-effective. [In one study] the points selected included ST-36 (*zú sān lǐ*), SP-6 (*sān yīn jiāo*), and LI-11 (*qū chí*). The measure of insulin for each person was not over 16 units daily, or about 28.5% of what a comparison group used. The quantity of sugar employed was also correspondingly reduced. They also tried injections on SP-15 (*dà héng*), and on ear points, and found that effectiveness was not noticeably decreased.

In Fu Zhou, a combination of ear points and body points were used with insulin injection therapy on 509 cases of schizophrenia. Those cured or markedly improved comprised 70.5%; the effectiveness rate reached 92.3%. [These studies indicated that] acupuncture-point injection therapy saves on medicine while improving the therapeutic results. It has thereby made the first small steps toward resolving the difficulties in medium- and long-term insulin therapy.

[In recent years,] drugs such as chlorpromazine have secured a growing role in psychopharmaceutical therapy for schizophrenia because of their convenience and low cost. However, it is not possible for them to completely replace the use of insulin and ECT, and furthermore they manifest pronounced side effects and require heavy dosages and prolonged treatment periods as well. Thus, an essential question addressing treatments for schizophrenia is how to reduce dosages without interfering with the therapeutic results. Experience shows that using electric stimulation on acupuncture points solves this problem.

When [researchers in] He Nan and other places added electroacupuncture on ear points to treatments that were being done solely with psychopharmaceutical sedatives, although dosages of medications were reduced, the effectiveness was enhanced. Daily dosages of chlorpromazine were reduced to 100-250mg. In cases where medication had been completed, but the illness was not completely resolved, auricular electroacupuncture also helped them achieve distinct improvements.

In short, acupuncture and the related therapies applied to acupuncture points are not only able to obtain good results for treating mental diseases when used alone, they are also able to improve on the shortcomings of the three major treatment methods used in mainstream psychotherapeutics. This combination brings out the best in both modalities.

In recent years there have been great developments in the different styles for applying acupuncture. Besides traditional body acupuncture, there are also [techniques of] five-person acupuncture, large needling (spine needling) therapy, electroacupuncture, auricular acupuncture, scalp acupuncture, fluid injection therapy, acupuncture suture-embedding therapy, point grasping and cupping, vessel pricking, and laser therapy. These new developments in the delivery of acupuncture have all been used with varying degrees of effectiveness in treating schizophrenia.

2. BODY ACUPUNCTURE THERAPY

[Researchers in] Shanghai took this saying from the *Inner Canon:*

> *Excellent acupuncturists will induce yang from yin, and induce yin from yang.*

They accepted adjusting yin and yang as their primary principle for deciding therapy. When they treated mania type diseases, they selected [points of] the conception vessel to induce yang from yin. They used GV-26 (*shuǐ gōu*) joined to GV-28 (*yín jiāo*), as well as PC-5 (*jiān shǐ*). When treating withdrawal disease they used the governing vessel, and thereby induced yin from yang; they selected M-HN-3 (*yìn táng*) joined to *xīn qū,*[12] and PC-6 (*nèi guān*).

For combined withdrawal and mania patterns they would choose one or two essential points from both the conception and governing vessels, and thus correct yin and yang for the entire body. They would also respond to developments in the patient's condition, and add one or two points from the five transporting-*shū* points, the source points, or the connecting-*luò* points of the related channels. For example, for heart qi inhibition, or feeble-minded and stagnant heart and spirit, the supplement was HT-5 (*tōng lǐ*). For effulgent liver fire with irritability, anger, and

---

[12]Translator's note—point *xīn qū* is located on the bridge of the nose, where a line connecting the two inner canthi would intersect the midline. This point combination is a family tradition from Dr. Jīn Shū Bái, an elderly doctor from Shanghai who has vast experience in treating mania-withdrawal with acupuncture.

cussing, LR-3 *(tài chōng)* was drained. For fearful patients with insufficiency of liver yin, KI-3 *(tài xī)* was supplemented, or SP-6 *(sān yīn jiāo)* was added to regulate yin. For dietary irregularity, the connecting point of the stomach, ST-40 *(fēng lóng)*, was added.

In Shen Yang, acupuncture with no other therapy was used to treat 403 cases of schizophrenia. Complete cures and obvious improvements occurred in 72% of the patients, and the effectiveness rate reached 88.5%.

For the group of patients who had agitated mania, the primary points used were: GV-14 *(dà zhuī)*, GV-26 *(rén zhōng)*, GV-18 *(qiáng jiān)* with a downward transverse needling to a depth of two to three *cùn; tóu niè* (located one cùn posterior and superior to M-HN-9 *(tài yáng)*, level with the top of the ear, located upon the temporal muscle where there is a protrusion when one bites down), and GV-24 *(shén tíng)* with transverse needling directed toward the posterior to a depth of two to three *cùn*.

For the group of patients with melancholia, the primary points used were CV-14 *(jù què)*, CV-17 *(dàn zhōng)*, Alert Spirit Quartet *(sì shén cōng)*, or M-HN-1, with transverse needling for two to three *cùn;* and CV-12 *(zhōng wǎn)*, GV-20 *(bǎi huì)*, and PC-5 *(jiān shǐ)* joining to TB-6 *(zhī gōu)*. For the group of patients with delusions, the primary points were CV-12 *(zhōng wǎn)*, CV-17 *(dàn zhōng)*, GV-24 *(shén tíng)*, CV-14 *(jù què)*, and GB-13 *(běn shén)*, with transverse needling directed toward the superior, for a distance of two to three *cùn*. Frequently used symptomatic points were [as follows]:

Auditory hallucinations	SI-19 *(tīng gōng)*, TB-17 *(yì fēng)*
Visual hallucinations	BL-2 *(zǎn zhú)*, M-HN-6 *(yú yāo)*
Fear	BL-19 *(dǎn shū)*, BL-15 *(xīn shū)*
Refusal of food	LI-4 *(hé gǔ)*, ST-36 *(zú sān lǐ)*
No speech	M-HN-21 *(shàng lián quán)*, GV-15 *(yǎ mén)*
Feeblemindedness and stupor	M-UE-1-5 *(shí xuān)*, KI-1 *(yǒng quán)*
Women with tendency to relapse during menstruation	premenstrual needling of CV-4 *(guān yuán)*, SP-6 *(sān yīn jiāo)*

Treatments were given once daily with 15-20 treatments comprising one course. For patients who at first did not cooperate with needling, treatments were enhanced with small dosages of sedative drugs. Usually chlorpromazine was used in doses not over 200g per day, or perphenazine was used in doses not over 10g per day. Once the patients accepted needling, the drug dosages were reduced or discontinued, depending on circumstances. When analyzing the relationships amongst all of the influencing factors, statistical methods showed that difference in sex, age, and frequency of disease occurrence had no apparent affect upon therapeutic results. However, when there was rapid onset and short duration of disease (less than one year), as compared to slow onset and prolonged duration of disease (more than one year), there was a pronounced difference.

3. FIVE-PERSON ACUPUNCTURE THERAPY

This therapy uses strong stimulation simultaneously [administered by five therapists] on multiple points. Five points are chosen for each treatment, including one point from each of the four limbs, and a head or face point. Examples of such points are: N-HN-32 *(dìng shén)*, GV-20 *(bǎi huì)*, PC-6 *(nèi guān)*, TB-5 *(wài guān)*, ST-36 *(zú sān lǐ)*, SP-9 *(yīn líng quán)*, and GB-34 *(yáng líng quán)*. A thick needle is used for a long time period (20-30 minutes), with a wide arc and rapid rotation, as well as lifting and thrusting. Or, one can connect a relatively strong electric current, and stimulate for 1/2 hour. This is done 2-5 times every day, or else needles are retained for 4-8 hours. According to reports, the success rate has reached 98.3%.

One can also use moxibustion, selecting from points GV-20 *(bǎi huì)*, PC-5 *(jiān shǐ)*, LR-1 *(dà dūn)*, SI-16 *(tiān chuāng)*, and HT-7 *(shén mén)*. Normally [this method] is used on schizophrenic patients who exhibit a vacuity pattern. Use seven cones of mugwort moxa on each point, and treat one time each day.

COMMENT

There are few reports on the use of traditional acupuncture (body acupuncture) for treatment of schizophrenia; articles about moxibustion therapy are even more rarely seen. These topics await more diligent future research. Five-person acupuncture therapy is a new procedure that has developed from the basis of traditional acupuncture. Its drawback is that the stimulation is very heavy and most patients are not receptive to it. Moreover, as many therapists are required, applying this therapy has definite drawbacks.

4. LARGE NEEDLE (SPINE NEEDLING) THERAPY

Large needle therapy, or spinal needling therapy, is a method that was used at Hospital 191 on point GV-16 (*fēng fǔ*) for treatment of schizophrenia. As time passed, other hospitals developed variations on this treatment; besides GV-16 (*fēng fǔ*), they also used points such as GV-14 (*dà zhuī*), GV-13 (*táo dào*), GV-4 (*mìng mén*), and GV-1 (*cháng qiáng*). Others selected supplementary points, such as TB-21 (*ěr mén*) for auditory hallucinations, and LU-8 (*jīng qú*) for frantic worrying. Some also used GV-20 (*bǎi huì*), combined with GV-1 (*cháng qiáng*) to treat symptoms such as psychological motor excitement.

When using large-needle therapy for treating schizophrenia, it is most suited for paranoid, hebephrenic, and mixed types, but it should be combined with psychopharmaceutical sedative drugs. The effectiveness rate has reached 98.7%, or 30-40% higher than using only chlorpromazine. The insertion method is to use a thick, large, stainless steel needle, and insert it on the midline of the back or neck into soft tissue. A relatively deep puncture is required.

COMMENT

One must take great care to avoid mistakenly needling into the occipital foramen magnum, or canalis vertebralis, which would cause injury to the medulla oblongata or the spinal cord and create undesirable results. If a mistaken puncture occurs, some patients can fully recover, while others retain sequela, and some can even die. This should elicit great concern.

5. ELECTROACUPUNCTURE

Electroacupuncture therapy for schizophrenia already has broad clinical use, and achieves a relatively good result. Normally, at each treatment 1-2 pairs of points are chosen. 28 gauge 1-1.5 inch stainless steel needles are used with any model of electroacupuncture machine. Usually a continuous wave is used with a frequency of around 120 waves/second. The strength of stimulation is divided into strong, medium, and weak.

Strong stimulation (employing electroacupuncture for ECT using acupuncture points), means using the largest output of electricity. The peak shock value is approximately 60-70 volts. Each time, electrical stimulus is administered for 10-30 seconds. Often it is used on points of the facial region, especially TB-17 (*yì fēng*), GB-2 (*tīng huì*), and other points around the ears. The strength of shock is also divided into light (where facial muscles have convulsive spasms), medium (where head and neck muscles have convulsive spasms), and strong (where the whole body is rigid or has convulsive spasms). The strength of shock, the duration, and the frequency are decided by the circumstances of the case.

Medium stimulation means a moderate degree of current. The effect on the body's vessels is a peak shock value of approximately 30-40 volts, with stimulation administered for around ten minutes.

Weak stimulation means a relatively weak output of electric current. Its effect on the vessels of the body is a peak shock value of 10-20 volts, with a duration of stimulus of 10-20 minutes. Schizophrenic patients are normally treated 2-3 times each day. When a patient is extremely agitated and excited, or stuporous, the frequency may be increased. If the case shows improvements then the strength of stimulation and number of treatments should be gradually reduced. Normally one course of treatment lasts 3-6 weeks.

Reports gathered from 14 articles, describing clinical treatments on 2937 patients, showed that effectiveness rates ranged from 62.8% to 95.9%. The methods included body acupuncture, ear acupuncture, and scalp acupuncture. The points were mostly selected by the combined principles of using local points and distal points of the same channel. When electroacupuncture therapy was supplemented with Western drugs, the combined therapies had an even better result. In one study, 698 cases of schizophrenia were treated, and patients were randomly divided into a group treated solely by electroacupuncture, and a group receiving electroacupuncture combined with small dosages of sedative drugs (such as chlorpromazine or tardan in dosages less than 200 mg/day). Compared to simply using electroacupuncture by itself, or drug therapy by itself, the therapeutic effectiveness of combined treatment was higher; moreover, the effects were superior.

Besides having a certain therapeutic effect on short-term cases, electroacupuncture also attains relatively satisfying results for long-term patients. A report analyzing 350 clinical cases showed that the treatments of electroacupuncture combined with small doses of sedative drugs had definite benefits for every type of schizophrenia.

The primary points chosen for electroacupuncture were bilateral TB-17 (*yì fēng*), bilateral SI-19 (*tīng gōng*), bilateral *tóu niè* (extra point), bilateral GB-18 (*chéng líng*), bilateral GB-15 (*tóu lín qì*), GV-20 (*bǎi huì*) paired with N-HN-32 (*dìng shén*) (located 1/3 of the distance from GV-26 (*rén zhōng*) to the lip), and GV-20 (*bǎi huì*) paired with M-HN-3 (*yìn táng*). Additional points were: PC-6 (*nèi guān*), LI-4 (*hé gǔ*), LU-11 (*shào shāng*), ST-36 (*zú sān lǐ*), LR-3 (*tài chōng*), KI-6 (*zhào hǎi*), and KI-1 (*yǒng quǎn*).

The ear points used were [ear] *shén mén*, endocrine/sympathetic, brain stem, and heart. Usually one pair of points is chosen and divided into positive and negative poles.

For excited, agitated patients, TB-17 (*yì fēng*), SI-19 (*tīng gōng*), and extra point *tóu niè* were used in alternation. TB-17 (*yì fēng*) and SI-19 have definite effectiveness on auditory hallucinations. For addressing refusal of food, reticence, and stupor, in addition to TB-17 (*yì fēng*) and the other points, one may add points of the four limbs with strong stimulation. Normally, combining the use of a sedative drug in suitable dosage will increase therapeutic effectiveness and consolidate the results.

In another project, researchers divided 182 cases of schizophrenia into four groups for comparative observations. Their results indicated that with the sole use of electroacupuncture, or electroacupuncture combined with Angelica Qi-Coordinating Decoction *(Dāng Guī Chéng Qì Tāng),* it is possible to reach the effectiveness rate of administering chlorpromazine by itself.

Other researchers used sedative drugs to treat schizophrenia. After enhancing the treatments with electroacupuncture on ear points, they were able to markedly reduce the drug dosages, while increasing the curative rate. Daily doses of chlorpromazine were reduced to 100-250mg. For patients with incomplete recovery after receiving drug therapy alone, electroacupuncture on ear points allowed them to make distinct improvements. The measure of electric current for ear acupuncture was gauged by what the patient could sense.

COMMENT

The sensation reported by the majority of schizophrenics who are treated with electroacupuncture is that after treatments the head and brain are relaxed as if a headband had been released. The effectiveness is most superlative in the hebephrenic and delusive types. If one compares the individual uses of electroacupuncture therapy to chlorpromazine, the effectiveness rates of electroacupuncture tend to be higher, and the results are seen more quickly. Electroacupuncture therapy in schizophrenia can replace electric shock therapy to a certain degree. It carries no harm for the patient's memory, and can eliminate side effects such as cerebral dementia and memory reduction in patients who would otherwise receive ECT and large doses of sedative drugs.

Because schizophrenics are often unable to cooperate with treatment, during treatments one must act to prevent the following list of mishaps.

1. Due to lack of cooperation by the patient, beware of bent or broken needles.

2. At times when strong stimulation is used, the patient's masseter muscles can have a strong, sudden contraction. A patient could easily bite off their tongue, bite into a lip, or damage teeth. Therefore, before applying an electric current, first instruct patients to firmly clench their teeth. A physician can firmly grasp the patient's lower jaw. When current is increased it should be done steadily and slowly. Alternatively, one may place a cushioning substance between the patient's upper and lower molars.

3. When points such as TB-17 (yì fēng) and SI-19 (tīng gōng) are used with strong stimulation, one must pay close attention to prevent fainting from fear, cardiac arrhythmia, and stoppage of the heart organ. Thus, when using strong stimulation the current should not be on for too long, and periods between shock should not be too short.

4. When points of the line from TB-17 (yì fēng) to GV-16 (fēng fǔ) are used and needles are directed towards the center, normally the depth of needling should not exceed 1.5 cùn. Overly deep insertion can cause the needle to enter the cerebral marrow or the medulla oblongata, and create unintended results.

5. When selecting points on the midline, such as GV-20 (bǎi huì), paired with either Spirit Stabilizer (dìng shén), Hall of Impression (yìn táng), or M-HN-21 (shàng lián quán), electric current used with strong stimulation can easily set off an epileptic type of grand mal. When using the points tóu niè or GB-18 (chéng líng), occasionally a similar response may occur. For that circumstance one should manage it as an epileptic seizure.

6. When using strong stimulation on TB-17 (yì fēng), SI-19 (tīng gōng), and other points around the ear, the patient may hold his breath. If the period becomes prolonged, the patient's face may turn green, or purple, or show other signs of oxygen deficit, and unintended results may occur. Thus, when doing strong stimulation one should pay close attention to the patient's face, and reduce the quantity of current in due time in order to avoid undesirable consequences.

7. For patients with cardiac disease, pulmonary disease, bronchial asthma, organic pathological developments of the brain region, high fever, or broken bones, as well as old and feeble patients, normally it is not suitable to do electroacupuncture therapy with strong stimulation on points of the head region, points around the ear, or ear points. However, weak or moderate stimulation may still be used.

It should also be noted that when using acupuncture therapies for schizophrenia, due to variations in types, circumstances of the illnesses, and degree of development, there can be a great disparity in treatment effectiveness. But no matter what type, all require persistence over a long period of therapy. After the main symptoms have been ameliorated, one should still treat for a period of time in order to consolidate the therapeutic results.

Over recent years a great variety of acupuncture therapies have been used in the treatment of schizophrenia. [Current research follows the theory that] points of the four limbs may not be ideal in their therapeutic results, whereas points closer to the cranium produce a higher curative rate.

6. AURICULAR ACUPUNCTURE

When auricular acupuncture is used to treat schizophrenia, it can reduce the dosages of sedative psychiatric drugs, as was explained above. Moreover, auricular acupuncture has reached a 94% success rate in treating auditory hallucinations, and catatonic stupor, while it has a relatively poor result on melancholia, delusions, and chronic schizophrenic disorders. One may select points based on symptomatology or on pattern identification. Some people use pulsating electric current on ear points and do not needle.

COMMENT

When performing treatment with auricular acupuncture, it is not suitable to use too many points. Normally 1-2 points are considered few, and 3-5 points are considered many. When it is necessary to do daily treatments, or to treat continuously and frequently, it is best to needle one side per treatment, and alternate from side to side. When doing electroacupuncture on ear points the electric current cannot be exceedingly large, and the length of time cannot be prolonged.

7. SCALP ACUPUNCTURE

The theoretical foundation of scalp acupuncture is that regions on the surface of the head or scalp correspond to regions of the cerebral cortex. When one needles on the regions that correspond to the cerebral cortex regions, it affects the focus of disease in the representative region of the cerebral cortex, and thereby achieves the aim of treatment. By extension of this concept, differing point regions have been established on the scalp. There is a cranial surface region, a functional region, a psychological symptom region, a psychiatric symptom mixed with gyrus function region, and also a brain lobe region. When needling in these regions, apply rotation manipulation or else use electric current stimulation. For visual and auditory hallucinations and delusions, the results are very good.

In Nanjing, scalp acupuncture was used on 296 cases of schizophrenia with hallucinations. The primary points were GV-19 (*hòu dǐng*) joined to GV-20 (*bǎi huì*). Additional points added relative to specific symptoms included:

Visual hallucinations	Join GB-17 (*zhèng yíng*) to GB-16 (*mù chuāng*)
Auditory hallucinations	Join TB-19 (*lú xī*) to TB-17 (*yì fēng*)
Gustatory hallucinations	Join GB-11 (*qiào yīn*) to BL-10 (*tiān zhù*)
Olfactory hallucinations	Join BL-6 (*chéng guāng*) to BL-5 (*wǔ chù*)
Haptic hallucinations	Join BL-7 (*tōng tiān*) to GB-17 (*zhèng yíng*)
Vestibular hallucinations	Join GV-16 (*fēng fǔ*) to BL-10 (*tiān zhù*)
Visceral hallucinations	Join GB-11 (*qiào yīn*) to TB-19 (*lú xī*)

Use transverse insertions to join points or to join channels. Employ rotation manipulation, as well as shaking-needle manipulation methods. After obtaining qi, quietly retain the needles for

1-3 hours. Treat once each day, with ten treatments considered the first course. Continue a second course with treatments administered every other day, for ten more treatments. For a third course, do acupuncture two times each week for a total of ten more treatments.

Results show that the effects are best in patients who improve during the first course of treatment, while those who show results in the second course of treatment have the next best result. If after three courses of treatment there is no benefit, one should adopt another modality. There is no clear relation between therapeutic effect and duration of disease. The overall effectiveness rate in the original trials reached 96%.

COMMENT

Scalp acupuncture is safe to apply and is without side effects. Scalp acupuncture treatment is especially noted for making a rapid and lasting result for schizophrenics with hallucinations. In addition, scalp acupuncture is quite suitable for treating neurosis. [It should be noted that] the theoretical basis of scalp acupuncture and its correspondence to regions of the cerebral cortex await further advances in research.

8. FLUID INJECTION THERAPY

Fluid injection therapy, also called point injection therapy, is a unique medical procedure. Its foundation derives from the theories of therapeutic point and channel stimulation from Chinese medicine, combined with the theories of Western pharmacology and injection methods from modern Western biomedicine. It has the combined therapeutic effects of both drugs and channel-point capacities.

The points commonly used for fluid injection therapy are the same as those used in body acupuncture. The drugs employed vary from hospital to hospital, and for different types of patients. For excited type patients [use] 0.2% chlorpromazine, 0.3% tardan, 10% *angelicae sinensis radix* (*dāng guī*) injection fluid, or 5%

spiny jujube (zǎo rén) injection fluid. For melancholic type patients [use] either placenta tissue fluid, or 0.3% angelica sinensis radix (dāng guī) injection fluid. At each point 0.5-1.0ml is injected.

Researchers in Jiang Su, Beijing, and other places used the formula Fú Mán Jiān[13] [consisting of] dried/fresh rehmannia [root] (shēng dì), ophiopogon [tuber] (mài dōng), atractylodes [root] (bái zhú), acorus [root] (chāng pú), dendrobium [stem] (shí hú), moutan [root bark] (dān pí), root poria (fú shén), tangerine peel (chén pí), mutong [stem] (mù tōng), and anemarrhena [root] (zhī mǔ), with additions and deletions. It is manufactured into a fluid for acupuncture point injections, and is an outstanding treatment for schizophrenia patients who have relapses during periods of remission.

Other practitioners have injected 1% phenol-water solution into points of the sacro-coccyx region, reaching an effectiveness rate of 83.3% Others injected Vitamin B1 or B12 into points of the ear region combined with small dosages of Western drugs for mental disorders and had a very nice result in treating auditory hallucinations. Other researchers injected 10mm of placental tissue fluid into points such as BL-10 (tiān zhù) and GB-20 (fēng chí), and this treatment alone corrected auditory hallucinations and delusions. As injecting insulin was mentioned earlier, we will not review it here.

COMMENT

Fluid injection therapy is relatively easy to perform. There is no particular discomfort, and the length of needle retention is shorter than in traditional acupuncture. But there are still numerous questions that await resolution. For example, understanding how we should choose medicines for injection, fix quantities of dosages and concentrations, and research point formulas combined with prescription choices, as well as discovering a clear explanation of its mechanism, would clarify the indications and

---

[13]Translator's note: The name "Fú Mán Jiān" is similar to a trade name. The translation could be rendered as "Wildness Treating Tea," but it is not a formula that one would find by this name in reference books of TCM formulas.

parameters. [It should also be noted that] points located on the hands, such as LI-4 *(hé gŭ)*, should not be injected with strongly stimulating drugs, in order to prevent accidents.

9. ACUPUNCTURE POINT SUTURE-EMBEDDING THERAPY

When this method is used for schizophrenia, normally there is embedding of a "0" gauge, 1.5 cm. length suture in acupuncture points of the auricular region, or in points of the governing vessel, such as GV-15 *(yă mén)*, GV-14 *(dà zhuī)*, or GV-13 *(táo dào)*, and other such points. Normally 2-4 points are used in each treatment, with 1-2 treatments per week, and ten treatments comprising one course.

At some hospitals, when sutures are embedded, they also use electroacupuncture and small doses of chlorpromazine, as this can improve the effectiveness. Suture embedding therapy has a distinct effect on schizophrenics who exhibit confused behavior, unsteady emotions, delusions, and linguistic or genuine hallucinations. For chronic schizophrenia, especially for psychomotor retardation, the success rate has reached 94.1% However, another researcher has reported that it is ineffective for schizophrenic thought disorders.

COMMENT

Embedding sutures on acupuncture points is a modern form of therapy that creates a continuous weak stimulation. In one course of therapy there may be embedding done at 10-20 points, and the sutures embedded may total 15-30 centimeters. The subdermal tissue is not able to absorb this kind of foreign body in a short period of time. Therefore, during administration one must strictly sterilize to prevent infection. If fainting, nausea, or local pain and swelling occur, one may give a hot compress or warming moxibustion. Although sometimes such developments abate on their own, one must maintain close observation.

10. POINT GRASPING AND CUPPING THERAPY

There are also reports of using point grasping and cupping to treat schizophrenia. In point grasping, the fingers are pressed heavily on heart, lung, and kidney *shū* points, as well as others. There is also rapping on GV-4 *(mìng mén)* and afterwards cups are attached along the bladder channel in the dorsal region, moving from above to below. Four cups are attached on each side, and the cups remain in place for 1/2 hour. Next, extra point *ān níng* is pinched and grasped.[14] SP-15 *(dà héng)* and mental sedatives are used as well. This method has had a reported success rate of 91.68%.

In addition there is a report of using incision treatments and cupping therapy for treatment in 162 cases of schizophrenia, with an overall success rate of 96%.

METHOD OF TREATMENT

Incision cupping locations are divided into four groups in the dorsal region, along the governing vessel and the *huá tuó jiā jǐ* points. Incisions are made to a depth just below the dermis (2-3mm). Immediately after making the incisions, cups are attached two times, each time for 6-8 minutes. The first time, 10-30ml of blood fluid is suctioned out, while the second time, a scant measure or even no blood emerges. After removing the cups, Yunnan White *(Yūn Nán Bái Yào)* is applied over the incision and the skin covered by the cup; this is done in order to staunch bleeding, dissipate stasis, and prevent infection. Next a layer of gauze is securely taped to the top. The four groups are done in order from top to bottom. At each session, incision and cupping is done on one group, and every other week incision and cupping is done one time.

COMMENT

There are only isolated reports of using the above treatment for schizophrenics. Its mechanism awaits further research.

---

[14]Translator's note—*Ān níng* is located bilaterally on the lower third of the neck, at the location 1cm posterior to the pulsating point of the carotid artery.

11. VESSEL PRICKING THERAPY AND LASER THERAPY

For vessel pricking therapy the primary points are M-HN-9 (*tài yáng*) and LI-11 (*qū chí*), with supplementary points such as BL-40 (*wěi zhōng*) and ST-40 (*fēng lóng*). Pricking into shallow blood veins and vessels to let out a small portion of blood has reached an effectiveness rate of 70% in schizophrenics with repletion diseases, and with heat diseases.

Laser therapy employs helium-neon laser rays in place of needles to treat acupuncture points. For schizophrenics of the delusive type and with genuine auditory hallucinations, the results are relatively good. The success rate has reached 52%.

COMMENT

The number of reports regarding clinical use of these two methods are few in number; they await future advances and conclusions.

IV. PSYCHOLOGICAL THERAPIES FOR SCHIZOPHRENIA

Psychotherapy is a system of multiple methods to induce positive effects on the psyche. However, it principally functions through the use of language to explain, inspire, guide, help, and teach, in order to reduce or eliminate the patient's symptoms and sufferings, and advance the recovery of health. Psychotherapy for patients who retain self-awareness, or even those with no psychological declines, is still important. Psychotherapy is particularly useful after effective treatment.

Modern physicians must look seriously at the clinical applications of psychology. Some believe that psychotherapy is not only a basic method for treating psychological disorders but has practical uses in every field of medicine. It is clinically proven that if a doctor disregards or ignores the psychological state of a patient or says inappropriate things, he/she can often precipitously cause the effects of suggestions and self-suggestions, which may cause a patient's health to decline.

For example, there was a woman whose husband had died of cancer, who sought medical treatment for heart palpitations due to excessive grief. The doctor advised that if she did not loosen up a little, she might suddenly go crazy. This woman's work place was located near a residence for patients with mental disorders. Every day while going to and from work, she would see that residence and recall the doctor's phrase. After a time, the result was a bout of hysteria. This is a case of "suggestions by others" leading to illness.

Another woman had a relative die from a brain tumor, and always suspected that she was sick herself. As a result, she often had nightmares, did not want to eat or drink, and finally was unable to arise from bed. This is a case of "self-suggestion" leading to illness. Thus, in treating schizophrenia, keeping the patient's psychological state in mind is crucial.

1. WORKING TO GAIN THE PATIENT'S TRUST

Schizophrenia occurs in a multiplicity of types, with extensive variations. But the overwhelming majority share one common special feature: the patients greatly doubt or oppose the physician. Thus, a physician must be possessed of sincerity and sympathy, and have an attitude of service toward all aspects of the patient. No matter how peculiar the patient's state of mind is, no matter how impulsive the patient is emotionally, no matter how crude his or her behavior, one must maintain a steady dignity and receive them with consideration and sincerity in order to win their trust. Moreover, with the patience required for drops of water to wear holes in stones, one must encourage and assist a patient to fully express the troubles dwelling in their innermost heart, the conflicts in their thoughts, or the concrete problems in their life and work. Once able to express these troubles, a patient will feel much more at ease. This is a prerequisite for successful psychotherapy.

2. COMPETENCE AT OPENLY OBSERVING THE THOUGHTS AND FEELINGS OF A VARIETY OF PATIENTS

When someone suffers from a psychological disorder, there are definite internal causes. However, the occurrence of disease is most often related to life at home, to social activities, or to work-related events. Moreover, the elements that are the provoking causes of psychological disorders in homes and society are of astoundingly vast complexity. Thus, if a doctor wants to accomplish his aim, he must also be familiar with people from every class of society, including their lifestyle, customs, mental outlooks, and cultural backgrounds. A doctor should understand the special characteristics and accommodations entailed by the customary psychological responses of people from different locations, of different ages, and with different occupations. Only with a broad and deep understanding of society and people is it possible for effective communication with all manner of patients. Reaching a level of shared language with a patient is instrumental in assisting the patient to expose their true thoughts.

3. INITIATING WORK WHERE THE PATIENT IS ENGAGED

When doctors perform psychotherapy methods for mentally ill patients, they must guard against subjectivity, narrow focus, and over generalizing. They must adapt to each individual patient, and have a precise aim for helping the patient analyze and review symptoms to find the root source of their disorder. Afterwards, based on the special features and individual circumstances, they must practically and realistically plan an appropriate direction and suitable steps for resolving the problems. In particular, at the outset of treatment, one should initiate work with what most engages the patient, and overcome any estrangement between the physician and patient. The patient's faith in the doctor and the medical procedures, as well as in the overall therapy, should be cultivated.

For example, if the patient is a lover of ancient literature, then one might undertake [a discussion of] historical events, certain ancient poems, or parables to console them. If the patient is an aging laborer with no intellectual background, one might use a machine as a metaphor: explain that when a person is sick it is not necessarily true that a component is ruined; usually when the parts have flaws in their performance, once the breakdown is repaired the machine is able to work as always. If the patient is an old farmer, one might talk of raising crops. Waterlogged crops might be used as a simile for exuberant dampness in the human body, and droughts or dry spells as a simile for a human body suffering from depleted and reduced fluids. Likewise, dispelling dampness would approximate draining floods; enriching yin and increasing humors would approximate irrigation. In general, the procedure for performing successful psychotherapy on mental health patients is to select the right key for the right lock.

4. DEVELOPING AN ADAPTABLE STYLE

When performing psychotherapy on mental health patients, the main form of therapy is for the doctor to hold private conversations with the patient. This is because many patients do not wish to express their true feelings in front of people who accompany them (usually family members) or before strangers.

The atmosphere of the clinic should be tranquil, orderly, and clean. Usually the best time is after the patient has rested and is in full spirits. It is not suitable to do therapy in the evening, as during discussion the patient may explain experiences or psychological events that elicit emotional waves which could interfere with sleeping that night. Discussions should not be too long; normally about an hour is suitable with 1-2 days in between. For nervous and tense patients, sessions can be once per day. Each discussion should have a certain goal, and a planned agenda of contents. One should accomplish a good estimate of what can be done.

To help patients have a basic knowledge of psychology, and to relieve their worries and dispel misconceptions, a group therapy format is also appropriate. Usually group members share a similar kind of disorder, a close cultural background, and are in a period of recovery or improvement. After hearing the doctor's explanations, advice, and encouragement, some patients with evident improvement in their health are asked to introduce their personal history, that they may encourage and inspire other patients. This form of therapy can not only reduce the workload for medical staff, but more importantly it can utilize the mutual influences within the group to improve therapeutic results. Ten to fifteen people is a good size for group therapy, with sessions of about two hours. The frequency of discussions is set according to circumstances.

HYPNOTIC SUGGESTION THERAPY

As hypnotic suggestion therapy can easily cause delusions in schizoid patients, it should not be employed. Clinically, hypnotic suggestion therapy effectively treats patients with episodic hysteria. It should also be pointed out that recommending a long vacation or travel to the patient, with the intention of making the patient as happy as possible in order to avoid relapse, is often counterproductive to the aim.

V. OTHER MEASURES

1. CHINESE MEDICINAL AGENTS IN COMBINED THERAPY

In recent years, combining treatments for schizophrenia with Chinese medicinal agents as the major modality has resulted in satisfying therapeutic results. Clinical experience shows that this approach has the redeeming features of quicker cures, higher success rates, low relapse rates, and infrequent sequela. Moreover, there are already numerous kinds of medicinal agents with a high cure rate which treat schizophrenia cases that were previously unresponsive to treatment, or that had poor results.

In Beijing, Chinese medicinal agents were the primary therapy for 117 cases of schizophrenia, with a cure rate of 77.3%, and an over-all effectiveness rate of 98.2%. In particular, the doctors employed a combined therapy of Chinese medicinal agents, acupuncture, and small doses of chlorpromazine.

In accordance with the spirit of establishing treatments for identified patterns, the treatment principle for mania patterns was to course and drain, clear and rectify. Three formulas were selected to treat mania:

1. MANIA-TREATING QI-COORDINATING DECOCTION
(Zhì Kuáng Chéng Qì Tāng)

rhubarb *(dà huáng)*	30g
mirabilite *(máng xiāo)*	15g
Sichuan magnolia [bark] *(chuān pò)*	15g
hematite *(zhě shí)*	60g
perilla fruit *(sū zǐ)*	15g
coptis [root] *(huáng lián)*	15g
scutellaria *(huáng lín)*	15g
crude gypsum *(shēng shí gāo)*	60g

2. MANIA-TREATING HUMOR-INCREASING QI-COORDINATING DECOCTION
(Zhì Kuáng Zēng Yè Chéng Qì Tāng)

scrophularia [root] *(yuán shēn)*	30g
ophiopogon [tuber] *(mài dōng)*	24g
dried/fresh rehmannia [root] *(shēng dì)*	24g
crude gypsum *(shēng shí gāo)*	60g
anemarrhena [root] *(zhī mǔ)*	15g
rhubarb *(dà huáng)*	15g
mirabilite *(máng xiāo)*	9g

3. HUMOR-INCREASING MIND-STABILIZING DECOCTION
(Zēng Yè Dìng Zhì Tāng)

scrophularia [root] *(yuán shēn)*	30g
ophiopogon [tuber] *(mài dōng)*	24g
dried/fresh rehmannia [root] *(shēng dì)*	24g
crude gypsum *(shēng shí gāo)*	60g
anemarrhena [root] *(zhī mǔ)*	15g
scutellaria *(huáng lín)*	9g
coptis [root] *(huáng lián)*	9g
mutong [stem] *(mù tōng)*	9g
poria *(fú líng)*	15g
hematite *(zhě shí)*	30g
licorice [root] *(gān cǎo)*	6g

Withdrawal patients were treated with two formulas:

1. WITHDRAWAL-TREATING DEPRESSION-RESOLVING DECOCTION
(Zhì Diān Jiě Yù Tāng)

bupleurum [root] (chái hú)	15g
angelica [root] (dāng guī)	12g
white peony [root] (bái sháo)	9g
atractylodes [root] (bái zhú)	9g
poria (fú líng)	15g
cyperus [root] (xiāng fù)	9g
sparganium [root] (sān léng)	6g
rhubarb (dà huáng)	9g
barley sprouts (shēng mài yá)	15g
pinellia [tuber] (bàn xià)	15g
tangerine peel (chén pí)	12g
licorice [root] (gān cǎo)	9g

2. STASIS-BREAKING BRAIN-AROUSING DECOCTION
(Pò Yū Xīng Nǎo Tāng)

peach kernel (táo rén)	30g
carthamus [flower] (hóng huā)	12g
angelica [root] (dāng guī)	12g
dried/fresh rehmannia [root] (shēng dì)	15g
red peony [root] (chì sháo)	9g
ligusticum [root] (chuān xiōng)	3g
sparganium [root] (sān léng)	9g
zedoaria [rizome] (é shù)	6g
crataegus [fruit] (shān zhā)	9g
barley sprouts (mài yá)	15g
gizzard lining (jī jīn)	6g

In addition, Mania-Withdrawal *Luò*-Arousing Decoction (*Diān Kuáng Xīng Luò Tāng*), formulated by Wáng Qīng Rèn of the Qing Dynasty, was used.

2. ACUPUNCTURE IN COMBINED THERAPY

[In conjunction with the formulas listed above, use] GV-26 (*shuǐ gōu*); Beside the Tiger (*hǔ biān*)[15] joining to SI-3 (*hòu xī*); LR-3 (*tài chōng*) joining to KI-1 (*yǒng quǎn*); ST-36 (*zú sān lǐ*); LI-11 (*qū*

---

[15]Translator's note: Beside the Tiger (*hǔ biān*) is located medial and inferior to LI-4 (*hé gǔ*), 1.5 *cùn* from the metacarpophalangeal joint.

chi); and CV-12 (*zhōng wǎn*) were used as the primary points. At times of unquieted manic agitation, a four *cùn* needle was inserted at a 30 degree angle to directly join CV-13 (*shàng wǎn*), CV-12 (*zhōng wǎn*), and CV-10 (*xià wǎn*). The needle was retained until the patient was calm.

The major points for electroacupuncture were divided into 10 groups:

1. GV-26 (*shuǐ gōu*) and GV-23 (*shàng xīng*)
2. GV-26 (*shuǐ gōu*) and GV-20 (*bǎi huì*)
3. bilateral ST-36 (*zú sān lǐ*)
4. bilateral PC-6 (*nèi guān*)
5. bilateral LR-3 (*tài chōng*) joining to KI-1 (*yǒng quǎn*)
6. bilateral LI-4 (*hé gǔ*)
7. bilateral ear needles (Heart, *Shén Mén*, and Brain Stem)
8. CV-12 (*zhōng wǎn*) and CV-4 (*guān yuán*)
9. GV-15 (*yǎ mén*), and GV-14 (*dà zhuī*)
10. GV-15 (*yǎ mén*) and GV-26 (*shuǐ gōu*)

The Western drug used in accompaniment was chlorpromazine, given at 50-200mg per day. It was administered orally, by muscular injection, or by injection at ST-36 (*zú sān lǐ*). Normally the dosage did not exceed 150g per day. Chinese medicinal agents and acupuncture were given during the daytime, while chlorpromazine was administered at a set time in the evening. This method allowed both Chinese and Western treatments to exert their strengths, yet not mutually interfere. Analysis of the effectiveness rates revealed [the following]:

1. The lower the age, the higher the cure rate.
2. The shorter the duration of disease, the higher the cure rate.
3. Mania disease type had a higher cure rate than withdrawal type.
4. There was no marked difference in the effectiveness on patient gender.

In the city of Suzhou, researchers combined the treatments of an experienced and venerable Chinese physician with small doses of chlorpromazine to treat 146 recalcitrant cases of schizophrenia, and obtained fine results. Most of the patients had been taking standard therapeutic dosages of chlorpromazine, perphenazine, and other drugs for mental illnesses over a prolonged period, but with no effect or only poor improvement. The majority of patients had relatively long-term disease.

Within the 146 cases, the delusive type was most prevalent, with 114 cases. The treatment method was primarily to nourish blood and quiet the spirit, harmonize the middle and moisten dryness. Licorice, Wheat, and Jujube Decoction (*Gān Mài Dà Zǎo Tāng*) and Lily Bulb and Rehmannia Decoction (*Bǎi Hé Dì Huáng Tāng*) from *Jīn Guì Yào Luè* [consisting of the following ingredients] were combined in use.

treated licorice [root] (*jiǔ gān cǎo*)	10g
light wheat [grain] (*huái xiǎo mài*)	30g
jujube (*dà zǎo*)	5pc
wild lily bulb (*yě bǎi hé*)	10g
(dried/fresh) rehmannia [root] (*shēng dì*)	10g

For patients with pronounced psychomotor excitement, the additions were dragon bone (*lóng gǔ*) and oyster shell (*mǔ lì*); for pronounced hallucinations, lodestone (*cí shí*) was added; for pronounced delusions, the additions were spiny jujube [kernel] (*suān zǎo rén*) and silk tree bark (*hé huān pí*). For other conditions, medicinal agents were added symptomatically.

In 29 of the 146 cases, no Western drugs were used; the other cases required less than the recommended therapeutic dosages of psychiatric drugs. (Daily doses of chlorpromazine, for example, did not exceed 200mg/day.) The period of using Chinese medicinal agents ranged from 7 to 98 days, with an average of 16.8 days. The overall treatment effectiveness rate reached 81.4%, which is much higher than the effectiveness rate of chlorpromazine itself in treating schizophrenic disorders.

~ CHAPTER SIX ~
CONCLUDING REMARKS

SCHIZOPHRENIA IS A DISEASE of maladjusted brain function that arises from many sources. It is dissimilar to normal internal medical diseases, because loss of normal psychofunction occupies a major position in its clinical manifestation. This also forms its special nature for clinical diagnosis and prevention. Research into the uses of acupuncture and its various modernized forms during the past few years has steadily reached new depths. The curative effects are definitive, and clinical experiences are abundant. Laudably, acupuncture has demonstrated excellent prospects for utilization as a primary treatment for mental disorders. Because of this evidence, traditional assumptions have begun to change, and the possibilities for promoting development in this field are encouraging.

Besides broader clinical treatment and observation of schizophrenia, there has also been theoretical work performed to explore its basic mechanism. The following paragraphs summarize the various perspectives on the mechanisms by which acupuncture treats schizophrenia.

Some [researchers] believe that the effect of acupuncture activates reticular formation and cerebral cortex function. By adjusting the relation between the two, it promotes wakefulness of the cerebral cortex, while reducing the excess activity of the cortex, and also raising the strength of the sympathetic nervous system. Other researchers have thought that the basis of electroacupuncture is the same as with standard ECT methods. Electroacupuncture with a strong current shatters the dynamic structure of the nervous system so that the normal and pathological biophysical peculiarities are destroyed, which removes the inertia of a negative disease state. Afterwards, a positive excitement state reestablishes, and the disorder is cured. Medium and weak electric current has the effect of improving the states of either excessive inhibition or excitement, and allows the attainment of balance.

There are others who think that the effect of acupuncture needling on axons in the central nervous system is to strengthen and invigorate their transmission, modulating the function of the cerebral cortex and thereby improving or curing mental disorders.

Some people hold that from the perspective of biochemistry, electroacupuncture makes changes in the synthesis and distribution of the central nervous system. For example, as catecholamine increases, it affects mental activity and improves the state of a mental disorder.

Others feel that the effect of acupuncture reduces neurotransmitters such as noradrenalin within the brain. [Levels of] seratonin in the brain stem are also reduced. These changes then eliminate the state of mental disorder. Whereas assessments show schizophrenics usually have lowered levels of qi and blood, and because after treatments these levels usually rise, it is thought that one effect of acupuncture is to correct vacuity of qi and blood. Some observations clearly show that the phenomenon of qi radiation along the channels is higher in schizophrenics than in normal people. It is supposed that because the channels and connecting vessels have disharmony, that the effect of acupuncture is to harmonize the channels and network vessels. Emotional elements have been considered as a source of stimulation. Via a circuit from the hypothalamus to the pituitary to the adrenal system (the Selye system), internal enzymes develop changes that lead to chaotic metabolism and manifest as atypical mental activity.

The influence of acupuncture on internal visceral functions is apparent, and it displays correcting effects on the Selye system, which can correct mental disorders. Some researchers have observed that acupuncture needling in head and face region points, compared to points in the four limbs, cause larger electric wave strength and areas of influence in the brain. They surmise that points of the head region are more effective than points of other regions for correcting nerve activity. Other investigators have shown that points at relatively thin places on the cranium, on bone sutures, and close to blood vessels, have a better effect for treating schizophrenia than do points of other head regions.

During the last thirty years, both clinical and theoretical researchers achieved major advances in their studies. Although some work repeated previously-used methods, much of the content was refreshed. Whereas the mechanism of development in schizophrenia is quite complex, at present we are still in a research phase that influences a whole series of inquiries regarding rules and laws that demand deeper research and analysis.

According to research findings in the early 1980's by scholars in the psychology research center at Maryland University (USA), a person's birth date has a certain relation to at least one kind of mental disorder, and generally those who develop mental disorders in the early stages of life almost never have a family history of the disorder. They investigated a group of schizophrenia patients who corresponded to this type, and discovered that there were more than 35% more who were born in winter and early spring than those born in summer and autumn. Moreover, the number of patients born in December started to show a slight increase, while those born in January or early February were at the highest rate. By March a gradual decline had begun, while the number of patients with July or August births was the smallest.

However, this only speaks for statistics within a population of schizophrenics. If discussing the entire population, then the rate of winter-born people who have mental illness is still quite small. The causes of this wave in seasonal birth rates among patients can be explained in two possible ways: First, there may be a yet-undiscovered element that causes an injury to the central nervous system at the moment of or not long after parturition—an element that occurs in fluctuation with the seasons. Other possibilities are seasonally active disease agents, or dietary and nutritional forms of a seasonal nature. Second, influences during pregnancy can be suspected. It is also possible that those with a propensity to mental disorders have certain inherited traits that in spring or summer appear more frequently; thus, the rate of mental disorders is higher in members of the following generation who were in gestation during that period. However, these two theories still lack conclusive support.

In addition, Chinese and Western medical scholars presently do not have a singularly unified classification system for schizophrenia. The Chinese physicians' methods of pattern identification, and the Western doctors' differentiation of disease, are not yet unified on the basis of dialectical materialism. By reaping the special features from ancient and modern, from Chinese and Western, a new scientific method for differentiating types of schizophrenia can be established.

In sum, the mechanisms by which acupuncture treats schizophrenia, as well as the causes and development of schizophrenia itself, await more extensive research. In the encouraging light of advancing studies into the rules governing prevention and treatment, and with continuously improving cure rates, we should vigorously continue all efforts to attain further breakthroughs.

BIBLIOGRAPHY

1。黄帝内经素问，人民卫生出版社，1963。

2。灵枢经语释，山东人民出版社，1963。

3。晋。皇甫谧：针灸甲乙经，商务印书馆，1955。

4。宋。王执中：针灸资生经，上海科学技术出版社，1959。

5。明。杨继洲：针灸大成，人民卫生出版社，1955。

6。上海第一医学院《实用内科学》编辑委员会：《实用内科学》，人民卫生出版社，1973，1981。

7。南京神经精神病防治院：精神病学，江苏人民出版社，1960。

8。四川医学院等：精神病学，湖南人民出版社，1976。

9。张逢春：精神病治疗学，上海科学技术出版社，1959。

10。曹希亮：中医健身术，陕西科学技术出版社，1983。

11。田从豁等：针灸医学验集，科学技术文献出版社，1985。

12。陈家扬：实用中医精神病学，北京出版社，1985。

13。中医研究院：针灸研究进展，人民卫生出版社，1981。

14。李文瑞等：实用针灸学，人民卫生出版社，1982。

15。娄焕明等：精神分裂症发病因素调查—多元逐步回归分析，中华神经精神科杂志，（1）；40，1987。

16。郑延平：社会支持在精神紧张过程中的作用，国外医学（精神病学分册），（2）；91，1983。

17。王善澄等：精神病的心理应激问题，心理科学通讯，（1）；41，1985。

18。楼星煌：楼百层的针灸学术思想，中医杂志，（10）；51，1985。

19。秦德平：古代医家心理疗法验案选按，皖南医学院学报，（1）；48，1987。

20。张洪度等：金舒白老中医治疗精神病的临床经验，上海针灸杂志，（1）；6，1987。

21。史正修等：针刺治疗精神分裂症403例，辽宁中医杂志，（2）；41，1980。

22。张晨钟等：割，拔疗法治疗精神病，河南中医，（6）；46，1984。

23。王栋桥：以中医为主治疗精神病117例临床观察，北京医学，（2）；87，1980。

24。周长发：用程门雪老师的经验治疗146例"精分症"临床报告，上海中医药杂志，（9）；12，1982。

25。张鸣九：头皮针治疗幻觉296例的经验，中医杂志，（6）；52，1987。

INDEX

Am J Acupunct V. 125 #N6 1. 1997 pp 25-71
Comparative ~~study~~ clinical Study on the
treatment of Schizo with electroacupuncture
a reduced doses of antipsychotic Rys
~~Zhou you~~ Zhou gouy et. al.

They used:

Yintang (between eyes)(7 upper dantian
signified by curled white hair)

PC-7
PC-6   } all for
Ex-HN-5   } clearing heart fire